The Emergency Doctor's Guide to a Pain-Free Back

by Melissa Yuan-Innes, M.D.

M

The Emergency Doctor's Guide to a Pain-Free Back

*Fast Tips and Exercises
for Healing and Relief*

by Melissa Yuan-Innes, M.D.

Olo
books

Windtree
Press

This book is dedicated to you, the reader,
because you're actively seeking out ways to heal and
prevent back pain.

TABLE OF CONTENTS

INTRODUCTION

5 REASONS WHY YOU SHOULD READ THIS BOOK

You're probably reading this because you're in pain.

Eighty-four percent of adults get low back pain at some time in their lives.[1][2] So you and I are not alone.

(Wouldn't that make a great birthday card? *Happy 18th birthday! Party hard, because now you have an 8 out of 10 chance of hurting your back!*)

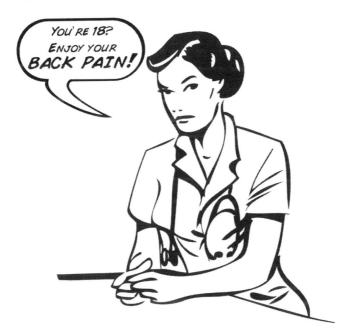

You picked this book because you want to fix your pain. You want relief. You want to heal this up. Now.

Well, like most doctors, I've got good news and bad news.

The good news is, most people do heal their backs on their own, without surgery, without an MRI or CT scan. Out of everyone who visits a doctor in the first three days of getting rocked by back pain, 9 out of 10 of them feel better within two weeks.[3] The fact that you're reading this means that you're motivated, which skews the odds in your favour.

The bad news is, I can't guarantee results. Note that I am *a* doctor, but I'm not *your* doctor, so all I can do is give you helpful advice on treatment and prevention. Even so, that puts you way ahead of everyone else who just pops pills and/or lies in bed for a month.

Let me introduce five ways this back pain book is different from other books.

1. I'm a doctor.

Most people who write books aren't medical doctors. (When I was in Los Angeles for an award ceremony, I gave my card to an actor who said, "Oh, are you some kind of New Age physician?" I laughed before I said, "No.") I spent decades in school so that I can dedicate my time to healing people.

2. I'm an *emergency* doctor.

That means I cut to the chase. I'm not going to lie to you so that I can sell you stuff. I'm not going to waste either of our time writing a long book that no one will finish. But because I'm keeping this book short and sweet, there may be times you want more detail.

That's why I created a special back pain destination on my website.

☆ Every time you see this star, it means that I've got bonus content for you at **http://melissayuaninnes.com/membership-join/**

To access that information, all you have to do is register with your name and e-mail address.

That will unlock videos, photos, checklists, worksheets and a whole cornucopia of information. The first video has practical tips on less painful ways to move when your back hurts.

3. I'll put results up front.

Most books start off talking about the author's credentials and give a crash course in anatomy. I already told you that I'm an experienced M.D. And frankly, I don't think most of you are interested in the nucleus pulposus. When you're in pain, you want relief, not a lecture. I will talk about anatomy later. But if you want to read it first, turn to the chapter titled <u>Anatomy</u>.

I'll start off with the history and physical exam, just like I would if I were seeing you in the emergency room, to point out some important details. But I'm going to cut to pain management and prevention pretty soon. So the information flow may seem abrupt. That's the ER, baby.

4. I know where you're coming from.

I'm not going to pretend I've got a white coat that magically protects me from back pain.

I've been you. Heck, I *am* you. Last Saturday, I killed my back. Not doing something glamorous like lifting a car off a helpless toddler and single-handedly resuscitating him. No. I woke up after hours of curling up in bed with my laptop, and I didn't want to move that morning.

Yup. I've been an emergency doctor for a dozen years. I've practiced yoga for almost two decades. And I still hurt my back.

I have to work 10 to 14 hour shifts, so when I'm in pain, I've got to turn it around fast. Within hours to days. Which is what I did for myself last week, and I'll show you how. Again, I can't guarantee identical results, because everyone is different, but I can point you down the right path.

5. I like to laugh.

Life is short. It feels longer if you read boring books. So I'm going to talk in my usual, informal way, making bizarre jokes, and if that offends you, just pick up one of those snooze books and have at it.

You're in pain. That sucks. Let's get started.

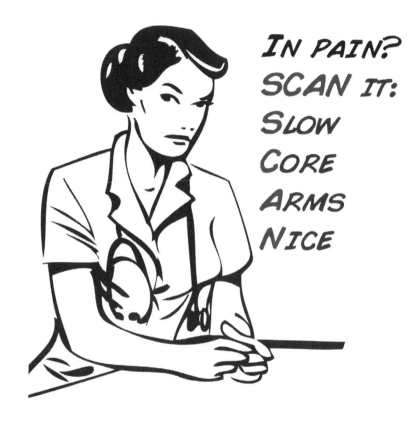

WHAT IF I CAN'T MOVE?

SCAN. SLOW-CORE-ARMS-NICE

Good news: for 97 people out of a hundred who go visit their regular doctor, back pain is *not* dangerous.[4] It hurts. It might hurt like @#%#@#^!!!!!! But severe pain does not equal severe spine/ nerve damage.

So it's safe to stir. You're not going to stay immobilized forever, unless you're dead. And you don't want that. Really. Even if it feels like it right now.

Pain-Minimizing Positions
You can recover by

1) lying on your side with a pillow sandwiched between your legs, or

2) lying on your back with your legs propped up on pillows or a chair. Less strain on your back. You can sleep like this, too.

But you want to keep bed rest to a minimum, usually limiting it to no more than one day.[5] The absolute best thing you can do is get moving as soon as you're able and get back to your normal life. That's what every study and guideline has shown for the past two decades.

Get Ready to Move
I want you to SCAN your body. **S**low. **C**ore. **A**rms. **N**ice.

1. Slow
Start off by moving slowly. And listen to your body.

It's like a traffic light. You used to be green, go go go! Right now, you're on the yellow, or maybe even red. So stop. Someone else literally has to pick up the kids or grandkids. You're not mowing the lawn or moving a piano today. Nope.

When pain-free, when you're back in the green, you can move fast again. But not now. Sorry.

When you're on red light (pain pain pain), find a comfortable position. After your back relaxes, slowly try to move again.

2. Core

Your back muscles need a break. That's why they hurt. Duh, right?

That means you have to use alternate muscle groups. Luckily, you've got a 3D group of muscles around your midsection: your core.

To find your core, lie on your back with your feet planted on the floor.

1. Place your hands on the lowest part of the sides of your belly and cough. Feel your transverse abdominal muscle working.

2. When you exhale, draw your belly button toward your spine and activate your back muscles.

3. Contract your pelvic muscles like you're stopping a stream of urine and holding in a bowel movement. Feel free to practice over a toilet.

Practice all three moves together, and you've got your core firing.

Your core is like a built-in belt or corset for you. Get it going, and your back muscles don't have to work as hard.

And guess what? When you're feeling better, I want you to make your core even stronger, to prevent back pain and sustain you during an attack. Yay!

3. Arms

Use your arms whenever possible.

Push up out of a chair. That's why they have arm rests and bed rails and even toilet rails.

Don't just lift yourself out of bed. Slowly roll on your hands and knees and push yourself up.

4. Nice

So many of us treat our bodies like machines. We're mad when they break. We want a refund. But guess what? This is your body. Unless you're living in 3020 and can get a body transplant, it's the only one you've got. So treat it like you'd treat your best friend, your pet, an innocent baby, or whatever gives you the warm fuzzies.

We don't talk about this much in medicine, but there's a mental component to pain, too. Depression and anxiety predispose you to back pain. Dr. John Sarno has built an entire industry talking about how repressed feelings cause back pain. I'm not that hard core. Yes, your body influences your mind, but sometimes, anatomically, something goes awry, and you need physical help.

Still, if you want your back to heal, it doesn't help to swear at it. Well, maybe that feels good for a second. But if you think of your back as strong, supple, and filled with vitality, it can't hurt—and it might help.

Be kind to your body.

Slow. Core. Arms. Nice.

You've got to shift, even if it's only to grab your pain pill. You know the song, "Move Like Jagger"? You want to move more like Jagger and less like jagged glass.

Even Jabba the Hutt shifted his eyes, tongue, and arm while lurking in his subterranean chamber. Let him be your role model.

TL;DR (too long; didn't read): move less jagged with Slow-Core-Arms-Nice.

☆ Log into my website at http://melissayuaninnes.com/membership-join/ to see the video about SCAN and photos of the pain-minimizing positions. I've also posted the SCAN cartoon.

On a blank sheet of paper, write down your own thoughts of how to add to the SCAN categories. How do you move slowly? How do you treat yourself nicely?

And if you've got your own moves you'd like to show off, please send me your tips, pics, or links to your videos.

WHERE DO I START?

HISTORY

Next, let's pretend you've come to see me in the emergency department.

I'll ask you the following questions, which are collectively called the history. Even if you skip the beginning of this section, please read the RED FLAGS at the end to gauge if you're at high risk for a serious cause of back pain. ☆ Then download a red flag checklist from my website so you can bring it to your next medical visit.

How did you hurt your back?

This is a chance for you to reflect on what trigger(s) you should avoid in the future.

Classic: you leaned over to pick something up, with your back hinged at the waist, and *ow!*

Reality: a minor injury set off your back pain. You lifted something and it bugged you a bit, but you kept working. Or you twisted to grab a wash cloth.

Did this happen at work? If it's a work injury, it means filling out paperwork for me. So tell me that up front.

When?

I want to know how long it's been going on. Usually, the triage nurse writes it down, but I have to check. If it's acute (short-term) pain, which generally means it's been going on for less than six weeks, 85 to 90 percent of you will get better on your own.[6] Your body will heal itself up.

That's different from chronic (long-term) pain, which people define as either more than six or twelve weeks of pain. I'm trying to cover both groups in this book, but acute and chronic pain are somewhat different animals, just so you know.

Where does it hurt? In the one spot, or does it go anywhere else (radiate down your bum or leg)?

The kind of pain that heads down your leg is commonly called sciatica, although some neurosurgeons get snippy and call it radicular pain. It's usually caused by an irritated nerve (more on that in the anatomy section).

Fortunately, this type of pain is less common. Most people still get better, but more slowly. A third feel much better in two weeks, and 75 percent are much improved at three months.[7] Even if you see a herniated disc on MRI, two thirds of the time, that disc heals on its own[8] [9]. Isn't that amazing, seeing the body heal itself? However, a 1998 study showed that one in ten sciatica patients at a specialist clinic will go for surgery, so that's still an option too.[10]

What makes the pain better? What makes it worse?

Usually your body will tell you what position works for you.

I come in the room and sometimes patients are standing up, saying, "Sorry. I can't sit down, or I'll never get back up." To which I reply, "That's fine. You do what you need to do."

Some people are lying in the bed, usually on their sides, with gritted teeth, afraid I'm going to move them.

The point is, they're already listening to their bodies. Even if it hurts. A plus.

Sometimes people say, "Nothing makes it better or worse." I don't believe that. You mean you'd feel equally good doing a back flip or wedged into a clown car? C'mon.

Pay attention to how your back feels depending on how you're lying, standing, sitting, and twisting your back, legs, or arms. Notice if it makes a difference, even a little bit, if you slap on an ice pack or get a massage.

I'm not inside your body. You are.

Ultimately, you're the one who's going to heal yourself. That means noticing what makes a difference.

Do you have weakness, numbness, or tingling?

I'm trying to figure out if you have nerve root compression. You can imagine that if a nerve is irritated, you'll feel a tingling or pins and needles as a warning signal.

Often, people say they feel weak "all over" from pain. But what I want to know is if you have weakness in your legs. Usually the problem is one-sided, although not always. And it's a bad sign if the weakness is getting worse. That would be a red flag. As is numbness around your genitals, bum, or upper thighs.

Did you try medication?

You'd be surprised how many people don't try over-the-counter medications at home. They think I want to see them in their original state. Actually, I don't. If they were in pain at home, they feel even worse after waiting in the emerg for five hours. So take something before you come in. And if you feel better and decide to wait for your family doctor, you just saved yourself five hours.

Have you hurt your back before?

Most people have. This may be the worst episode, but back pain is like the gift that keeps on giving. (Pain.)

Seventy percent of people relapse within a year. Luckily, your body will heal itself up again, much as it did the last time. But it can be like asthma, this low-grade problem that bugs you a little bit every day, but you kind of ignore it until it flares up every so often like a demon.

I like to know this in the emergency room, because odds are, if you have a history of neglecting back pain, you won't heal quite as fast. Unless you take it as a wake-up call to turn your life around and start working on prevention. The fact that you picked up this book is a good sign.

RED FLAGS

Now I'm going to go through the things I ask everyone to try and eliminate the dangerous conditions. Bad things are rare, but obviously I don't want to miss them.

1a. **Do you have trouble with your bladder or bowels today, meaning that you cannot pee *or* you're incontinent of urine or stool?**

1b. **Can you NOT feel the tissue paper when you wipe yourself? Or your upper thighs?**

1c. Do you have **worsening weakness in your leg(s)?**

In case you hadn't guessed, the dangerous answers are "yes."

What I'm looking for here is spinal nerve compression. It's very unlikely, but we do sometimes see it, particularly in cancer patients, and that *is* a medical emergency. We radiate the spinal cord to shrink down the tumour ASAP.

I have to say, in my dozen years of practice, only one person had signs of spinal nerve compression, and that was a patient who'd already consulted with a neurosurgeon. So it's rare.

The following answers are all normal: women who've had children often have stress incontinence (peeing inadvertently while jumping, running, coughing, etc.). Everyone's had diarrhea at some point, but it's usually not uncontrollable. People can feel their nether regions and bum when they're wiping them off.

Sometimes, people say, "Oh, yeah, I'm constipated!"

That's not diarrhea. That's the opposite of diarrhea. Constipation does tend to make back pain worse, because you're straining on the toilet. But it's not spinal nerve compression. High five!

2. **Do you personally have cancer?**

This follows on the last question. For most people, it's a no. Or "I used to have cancer, but I was treated ten years ago, and all my scans are negative." Or "My grandma had skin cancer."

What I'm looking for is an active cancer in your own body. Especially prostate, breast, lung or renal cancer that likes to attack the bone.

Sometimes people say, "Not that I know of." If they look skinny or tired, I might start asking questions about fatigue, weight loss, and so forth. But most people just plain don't have cancer. Which is good.

3. **Do you take steroids like prednisone?**

Some medications can thin the bones, and I need to know if you're taking them, because you're more likely to fracture a bone.

Of course, if you naturally have thin bones that tend to break, because of osteoporosis or osteogenesis imperfecta, I'll still check you for fractures.

4. Do you use intravenous drugs, like heroin?

I know this sounds fairly ridiculous, since it means I'm asking 80-year-old ladies if they shoot up, but I'm looking for abscesses (pus) on the spine. As you can imagine, shooting up with dirty needles makes it more likely that you'll seed bacteria in all sorts of unlikely places, including your spine.

In a developing country, or if you were homeless, I might ask about tuberculosis, which also enjoys attacking the spine.

5. Do you have a fever, chills, or weight loss?

Same as with number 4, I'm mostly looking for abscesses. Cancer can also give you a long-term, low-grade fever and weight loss.

6. Does the pain *never* go away, even at night, or when lying down?

We have to rule out cancer.

7. Do you have immune problems, like HIV or AIDS?

Abscesses again. Or other weird diseases. It just means I have to be more careful.

8. Did you fall, or get into a car accident, or anything like that?

You should already have told me how you hurt your back, but once in a while, I turn up stories about horrible car or construction accidents that a guy sustained in 1982. I'm mostly looking for recent trauma, but I'm interested in old injuries, too.

If you're over age 65 or have weak bones, I want to know about even minor injuries. I don't want to miss a fracture.[11] Which brings up another question…

9. How old are you?

I should already know this from your chart, but if you're over age 70, or even over age 50, you're more prone to fractures, infection, tumours, and aneurysms (weakened blood vessels).[12]

Children need special consideration. So if you're under 18, you should consult a different book. This one is aimed at adults with low back pain.

☆ Log into <u>my website</u> to get a red flag sheet to bring to your doctor.

A few more words about trigger incidents (the thing that set off your back pain)

"I sneezed." Or "I coughed." Sounds ridiculous, right, if that's what made your back hurt? It's embarrassing.

But actually, both of those things strain your back. So first of all, lean straight back, instead of torquing part of your body, and/ or brace yourself to sneeze or cough. A friendly tip.

And secondly, it's not like the most dramatic trigger story wins a gold medal. Usually, it's not one thing that sets off your back pain. It's a whole bunch of insults: didn't sleep enough, stress, slumping, too much sitting, and then—hey! One straw can indeed torment your back, if not break it.

Don't pay too much attention to the straw.

The straw is not important. If you obsess about it, you can delay your recovery.

Even if your straw was a life-threatening industrial accident where a ton of sheet metal fell on you—and I've heard some pretty scary stories—I suggest you work through what you need to (anger, grief, bargaining, filling out insurance forms, even suing, if you must) and then move on. You've got work to do. Over-dwelling on the past isn't going to help you.

All clear? Let's head on into the physical exam!

PHYSICAL EXAM

Let's get physical.

I want to examine you without hurting you too much.

As soon as I walk in the room, I'm checking how you look. Standing? Lying still because everything hurts (the usual position, which is actually reassuring that it's a muscle and bone problem)? Writhing in agony like you've got a kidney stone?

I'm looking at your vital signs, too, for a fever or a change in your heart rate or blood pressure. But mostly, I'm concentrating on a few areas.

1. Your back.

I run my hand up and down your spine. Is there one bony spot that hurts? I'm searching for fractures and abscesses while checking out your skin.

Is it more the muscles along one side, so you groan and say "that hurts" when I press on them? There's your diagnosis.

If your entire back hurts, that doesn't help me. Try to narrow it down if you can. You shouldn't hurt 10/10 (screaming, black-out levels of pain) over 100 percent of your back.

2. Your neurological exam.

You ask, "Do I have a pinched nerve? Is it my disc?"

Your body will help tell me. Often I'll ask someone to show me exactly where it hurts. Is it your back? Does it go down your leg, making it more likely that you have a disc problem? Do you have trouble feeling a light touch?

I'll check your reflexes and your strength, including the Babinski reflex where I run my nail along the bottom of your foot. Usually people say, "I can feel that," although one in a while, they burst out giggling or jerk their feet away.

As part of your exam, I'll do the straight leg test: you lie on your back and I'll lift your leg into the air, one at a time. I want to see if the pain radiates below your knee into the foot. Then I'll move your foot upward to see if the pain gets better or worse. I'd say less than twenty percent of people actually show nerve root impingement with this sign.

3. Your abdomen.

I need to rule out other causes of back pain. One we don't want to miss is a ruptured aortic aneurysm (the main blood vessel in your abdomen is leaking blood) More commonly, and very painfully, it could be kidney stones. But usually, people with a musculoskeletal cause hurt when they move, and that's the tip-off.

In a male child, I may examine the testes, which the boy usually finds hideously embarrassing, but can be considered part of a complete abdominal exam. Kids probably know if the pain is coming from their nether regions or not, but this is a just-in-case thing.

4. Rectal exam

We may save these for patients who have red flags and can tolerate a finger up the bum. I'm checking if you can feel the finger, if you can squeeze it, and, as a special treat for the guys, if there are lumps in the prostate. Moving on.

ANATOMY

BASIC ANATOMY

Here's what you already know: you have a spine, made up of bones. Spongy discs sit in between the bones, like shock absorbers. Your spinal cord runs inside the bones. Nerves stretch out to either side, so you can feel things on both sides of your body. It's actually very cool.

BONES, A.K.A. VERTEBRAE

Let's start with the bones. Do you ever hear TV doctors yelling, "We have to clear the C-spine!" or "Your problem is at L4-L5?" That's just medical shorthand for the cervical vertebrae (C-spine) and the lumbar vertebrae (L-spine).

I highlight C and L because that's where we usually run into trouble. The C(ervical) spine is your neck, so we check it after motor vehicle crashes, but that's a whole separate topic. The L(umbar) spine is the low back. That's what we're talking 'bout in *The Emergency Doctor's Guide to a Pain-Free Back*: low back pain.

The numbers correspond to the level. As you can see, the lumbar spine has five vertebrae. So if your doctors say, "You have a disc herniation at L4-L5," it means the disc is pushing out between your fourth and fifth lumbar vertebrae. No magic to it.

Some people do end up with problems at the T(horacic) spine and the sacrum, and the sacro-iliac joint (where the sacrum connects to the hips).

No matter where your pain is, I hope you appreciate the elegance of your spinal column, even in this simplified sketch. Looking good, baby.

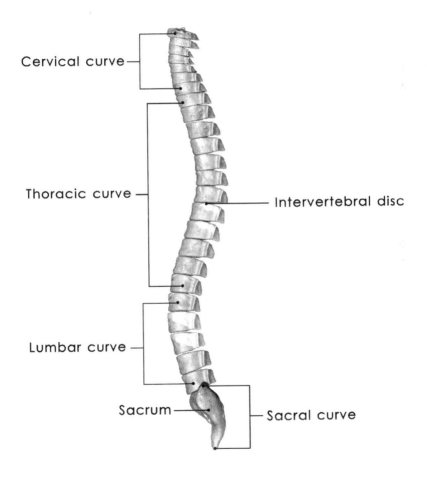

Cervical curve

Thoracic curve — Intervertebral disc

Lumbar curve

Sacrum — Sacral curve

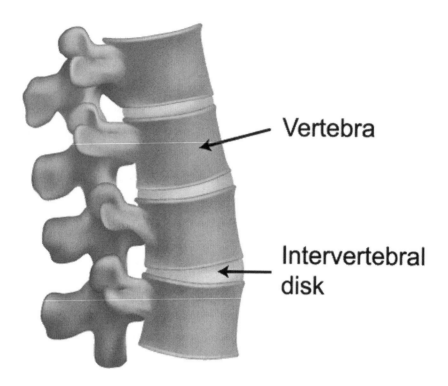

Vertebra

Intervertebral disk

INTERVERTEBRAL DISCS

You don't want your bones grinding against each other. That's where the intervertebral discs come in, sandwiched between the vertebrae to cushion them and add flexibility. Tall, healthy discs allow the spinal nerves to run off either sides of the cord.

You can think of the disc like an egg fried sunny-side up. The "yolk" is the *nucleus pulposus* made of collagen and water. The "white" is made up of *lamellae*, the layers of water and thicker collagen. Some doctors have also compared discs to jelly doughnuts, because the yolk is also like jelly. Yum-my.

Another cool fact: intervertebral discs are *avascular*. That means that instead of developing arteries and veins to circulate blood, they rely on osmosis—when you lie down, the water and nutrients can better diffuse in; and when you stand up, it helps push that waste out.

In other words, you've got to change positions and move around to keep the discs healthy.

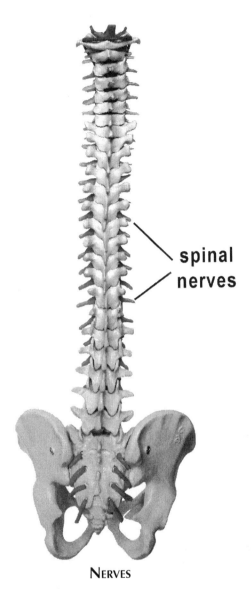

spinal
nerves

NERVES

I'm including the picture above not only because it kind of reminds me of a guitar, and because it's the first view as if you're standing behind the patient, but because it shows the spinal nerves, those little things poking out on either side, through the intervertebral foramen. (They've been cut off in this picture, instead of continuing out to the rest of the body, but you get the idea.)

Here's what you might not know: your spinal cord ends at the second lumbar vertebrae. So if you were secretly worried about getting paralyzed by low back pain, good news. A lot of the time, the pain is lower than your physical spinal cord. You're feeling your spinal *nerves*, not your spinal *cord*. A different animal.

Another important thing to know: the amount of pain doesn't correspond directly to the amount of injury. It just depends on your pain tolerance, which almost every patient or family member tells me is "incredibly high," just before asking for drugs.

Plus, you receive pain signals from a lot of places besides your spinal nerves. For example, the organs inside your belly, the muscles supporting the spine, or the *fascia* (Saran wrap around your muscles) can all give you a good one-two.

Muscles
Your body has a built-in weight belt/corset: your core muscles.

The absolute simplest definition of "core" is every muscle that stabilizes the spine. Therefore, every muscle from the neck down.[13] But that might be a little too broad, if it has you thinking, "Okay, now I have to use every single muscle below my head." And in fact, experts disagree on what exactly constitutes core muscles.

Let's focus on a few main groups that encircle your body, forming a 3D network of muscular goodness.

1. **Abdominal muscles**. Everyone wants the six-pack abs. But they're not the whole story, and working them too hard imbalances the body because you're concentrating on making a good-looking front instead of a stable back.

The visible abdominal muscles are the *rectus abdominis* and the *internal* and *external obliques*, the muscles that run vertically and somewhat diagonally (obliquely) on your body. And they are lovely and necessary muscles.

But you need the *transversus abdominis* (TrA), the deepest muscle that runs horizontally, and the only one that attaches to the spine, to really stabilize your back and hold your abdominal organs in like a corset before you start to move your arms or legs. It's the muscle on the right, labeled TrA in the next photo (supplied by Michael Teller[14]). If you're having trouble orienting yourself, the circle on the left is the belly button, so this is a shot of someone's left midsection.

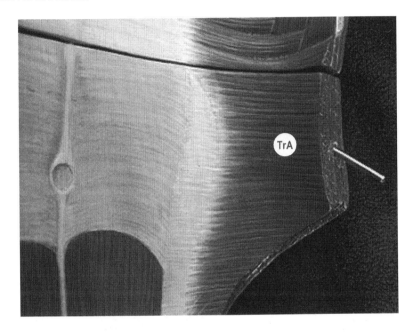

Here's a quick TrA finder exercise: slowly draw in your abdominal muscles. If you turn sideways in a mirror, it makes you look slimmer. (I used to do this when I was in my second trimester of pregnancy, to show off my "I look normal" vs "You can tell there's a baby in there" paparazzi views.) The deep muscles on both sides—away from your belly button—are working. You should also contract your pelvic floor, #5 in this list. Remember to breathe normally. Good times.

2. **Deep lower back muscles**. I like to think of the *erector spinae*, which literally means "keep the back upright," as your built-in mom telling you not to slouch.

We don't pay much attention to the *multifidus* in medical school, but they're little muscles that attach directly to the vertebrae and stabilize between different spinal levels. Small but mighty.

3. **Hip flexors.** You'd feel pretty sad if you couldn't knee someone in the crotch, right? Well, your hip flexors are the muscles you need to bend at the hip. They get tight if you sit for too long, which would be…all of the Western world, and maybe now the rest of the globe, too.

Your pals here include not only the crotch-busting muscles that flex your thigh like the deep-seated *iliopsoas,* and the more superficial and sexy thigh muscles like *rectus femoris, sartorius,* and the *tensor fasciae latae,* but you should also love your inner thigh muscles. The inner muscles of your legs stabilize your hips and pelvis and even the arches of your feet! So say thanks to your *adductor longus* and *brevis, pectineus* and *gracilis.*

4. **Gluteal muscles**. Not just for Kim Kardashian. Your rear end is your powerhouse.

For example, your *gluteus medius*: every time you walk and swing your weight from one leg to the other, you're saying hi to your glute med. If it's too weak, every time you swing your weight, the opposite hip will dip down.

5. **Pelvic floor**. You have to consider your pelvic floor, or else your body is like a wet paper box where the bottom falls out. With that charming image in mind, you might want to look up the *pubococcygeus* (PC) muscle and how to strengthen it: try stopping the flow of urine a few times, until you get a feel for it, and then you can build up your strength and endurance.

The main take-away is that the entire body is a well-calibrated system that works together beautifully, not to get bogged down in Latin names.

If you've got pain now, it's a signal that we need to move back to the balance and grace you were born with.

6 CAUSES OF BACK PAIN

1. MUSCLES

The most common culprit. You strained or even tore the muscles in your back. Happens to athletes, couch potatoes, weekend warriors...we all hurt muscles at one point or another.

Sometimes you can tell right away, oops, shouldn't have done that. Other times, you can't pinpoint the time or cause.

Muscles can go into spasm or cramp up. Although that may lock you in place and make you start swearing, it can protect the spine and prevent you from hurting yourself more.

2. SOFT TISSUE

Ligaments (which hold two bones together) and tendons (which connect muscle to bone) can get inflamed, pulled, or sheared off. Did you fall, get in a car crash, or lift something wrong? Did you try a sport for the first time in a long time?

If the ligaments aren't holding the vertebrae together right, your spine can't move properly.

And if the muscle's firing, but the tendon's not connected to the bone correctly, you won't move right.

Together, muscles and soft tissues probably account for about **70 percent** of back pain. "Lumbar strain" really just means hurting your back. This type of injury tends to heal up within six weeks.

3. BONE

If you've got bone pain, usually you can point to one very tender spot instead of the more spread-out soreness from a muscle.

Anyone can break a bone from a fall or other trauma. I know someone who tried to jump a ditch with a snowmobile and didn't make it. But you can shatter a bone much more easily if you have cancer, osteoporosis, or you're elderly. We also check for bone cysts, a tumour, or infection. Cheery thoughts, eh?

About **4 percent** of back pain comes from osteoporotic fractures.

4. DISCS

Ah, the intervertebral discs. The cushiony discs between the bones that can squish like a jelly doughnut. To further whet your appetite, Dr. Jack Stern compares them instead to fake crab meat, pointing out that both materials are a) flexible, b) made up of many different strands, which you can imagine pulling apart when torn by age or trauma, and c) don't have any blood vessels. The lack of blood supply makes it harder for them to repair themselves.

Remember, especially after age sixty, discs can and do bulge without pressing on any spinal nerves, which is called **degenerative disc disease**. The pain tends to centre around the middle of your back. It's worse if you stand up or if you're active, and it's better if you lie down. About **10 percent** of patients have disc degeneration or facet problems.

Disc herniation: if the disc's insides squish out and press on a spinal nerve, you can get pain running down your leg. It can feel like a stab of lightning. The pain might ease up if you bend that leg and get worse if you cough or sneeze. Some people get numbness or weakness in the leg, foot, or toes. Rarely, it can cause bladder or bowel trouble, one of the red flags that mean you should get to a doctor pronto.

Causes include injury and trauma, lifting something wrong, repetitive strain from activities, or age-weakened discs. Obesity and smoking also injure the discs.

If you've got **disc extrusion**, the squished-out bit no longer makes contact with the rest of the disc.

Only about **4 percent** of back pain patients have a disc herniation.

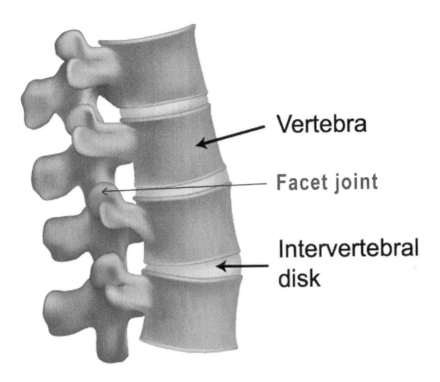

Vertebra

Facet joint

Intervertebral disk

5. FACET JOINTS/Z JOINTS

If you think of the vertebrae like Lego bricks locking into each other, the facet joints are the hook-ups in the back. If you like tongue-twisters, the more proper name is the zygapophyseal joints (Z-joints), but I'm going to stick to the more common name of facet joints.

When the discs start to wear down, these joints wear down, too, and get osteoarthritis.[15] [16] In 1927, Putti found facet joint arthritis in cadavers over 40 years of age.[17] I'm just throwing that in there because you can imagine how much fun that must've been, prying apart the backbones of 75 cadavers to look for signs of arthritis.

This is a tricky one to diagnose, though, because it can look like disc pain.

It can happen suddenly, like you leaned over to tie your shoelaces, and BAM. Locked up. Can't move.

The pain can radiate down to the bum, which seems like a disc, except it usually doesn't run past your knee and into your foot. It can get worse when you're straightening up, or leaning backwards, when you're riding in a car, or when you try to get out of a chair or sit up straight.

It hurts if you press on the facet joint, unsurprisingly.

And it can keep coming back.

Do you play tennis or golf? The twisting movements can set it off.

Because this one is harder to diagnose, you might need X-rays or a CT to look at the bones. Because it's a bony problem, an MRI isn't as good, although it will show you the discs and rule out problems there.

Sometimes the best way to diagnose this is by injecting the facet joints with a painkiller. The immediate relief tells you that was the right diagnosis.

Some experts think that facet joint pain doesn't exist in isolation. Other anatomical problems come into play, too.[18] It's estimated that degeneration of facet and discs together account for about 10 percent of back pain patients.

Some other helpful moves:

Sit on the edge of the chair.

Pelvic tilt: Tense your bum and tilt your pelvis forward. Do it several times a day.

Put a lumbar support in your chair, especially during a flare-up.

When you're standing, lift one leg up on a foot stool to relieve pressure in the back.

Plus the usual trial of nonsteroidal anti-inflammatory drugs (NSAIDs), if you can tolerate them, or heat or cold.

If nothing helps, you may get to the point where a doctor would kill the nerves to the facet joints by freezing them or burning them (facet rhizotomy). Or the last-ditch effort is a spinal fusion. I'll keep my fingers crossed that it doesn't get to that point for you.

6. NEURAL STENOSIS

Foraminal stenosis: is that what your MRI said? All that means is narrowing of the little tunnels where your nerve roots exit your spinal cord.

Spinal stenosis refers to the narrowing of the canal for the actual spinal cord. About **3 percent** of people have spinal stenosis.

In other words, your spinal cord or spinal nerve roots are being squeezed by bone. Sounds scary, but usually it just means that the bone hole is a bit smaller, yet *not* pressing on the spinal cord or roots, which is really the end point we're interested in.

This is something that happens over time, gradually. Arthritis, basically.

Spinal claudication from spinal stenosis: The more you walk, the more you get lower back pain, which means discomfort between your lower ribs and your buttocks that might radiate into one or both legs. The more you walk, the heavier your legs feel. They might start to wobble a bit. If you take a break, the pain eases up.

And if you bend forward, like over a shopping cart or on a bicycle, the pain also gets better. That's a hallmark of spinal stenosis.

Over the years, you get pain at shorter distances before you need to stop for a rest.

Your doctor will want to check the circulation and nerve conduction to your legs, because that can cause similar symptoms. (Public health announcement: almost always, when we diagnose people with bad circulation, a.k.a. peripheral vascular disease, they're heavy smokers. And vascular surgeons won't operate if you're still smoking. Yet another reason to butt out forever.)

What should you do?

Well, the first thing is to change your activities so they don't hurt so much. Like, if running or walking aches, but you can ride a bike for hours, the choice is clear.

And you can investigate different pain management options (oral painkillers, the possibility of epidural injections) with your doctor before you consider surgery. They're also investigating spinal spacers, which is basically inserting devices between your spinous processes, as well as more traditional spinal decompression surgery.

This is just a quick overview. I'm not pretending to cover every single source of back pain, but this is a useful way to categorize the causes.

If you'd like to read more about the categorization, check out Dr. Jack Stern's book, *Ending Back Pain*.[19]

If you want to read more about specific conditions that can cause back pain, turn to the section called <u>What does this mean?</u> It's a collection of diagnoses explained in simple ways.

I also realize that the numbers above don't add up to 100 percent, probably because we can't categorize all types of back pain. Which leads me to the next section, How to Feel Better, Fast.

HOW TO FEEL BETTER, FAST

GOOD NEWS: THE DOCTOR *DIDN'T* FIND ANYTHING

Most people don't have any red flags on their history or physical exam.

Let's assume you've got a new case of non-specific low back pain. More than 85 percent of the time, we don't find a particular cause.[20] That means, out of every ten people with back pain, for 8.5 of them, we can't immediately point to something and say, "That's it! Get rid of that bugger and you're done."

Guess what? That's *good news*.

You don't want me to find cancer, or a fracture, or an infection.

Because 97 percent of the time, it's a musculoskeletal (muscle, bones, ligaments, etc.) problem.[21]

So the vast majority of time, as much as it hurts, it's *not* serious.

Again, I recommend you see a doctor to make sure you fit into that 97 percent. But chances are, you do.

Which means you will *not* be paralyzed.

The pain *will* go away.

You *don't* need to pay tons of money to anyone reaching for your wallet for expensive tests or treatments.

Your body will heal itself.

Let's get started on the road to back to health.

HEALING TIPS BASED ON RESEARCH:

GRADE A, B, C

"Life is pain, Highness.
Anyone who says differently is selling something."
—Westley in William Goldman's *The Princess Bride*

I want to tell you the truth in this book. That means I'm trying to base my words on research instead of theoretical B.S. that fits with whatever expensive treatment I can auction off.

SHORT VERSION:

Grade A evidence: Try this. We've got good evidence that backs it up.

Grade B: Will probably help you. Research leans this way.

Grade C: Some studies say yes, some studies say no, or the studies were poorly-done.

LONG VERSION:

Back pain research is confusing. First of all, a lot of treatments, especially alternative/complimentary/integrative treatments, don't have any experimental evidence at all. In other words, they're not proven.

Someone says, "Drink pink vovo berry juice* for your back pain! It has twelve antioxidants and five flavonoids, and is high in vitamin C!" Someone in Florida posts online, "I drank it! My back is 100 percent better!" and soon you have a cult of a hundred, a thousand, a million people celebrating pink vovo berries. Pink vovo berry farms spring up next door. The paparazzi take pictures of Jennifer Aniston sprinkling organic pink vovo berries on her cereal, but no one ever actually did a study on vovo berries.

Thanks to the placebo effect, about 30 percent of people will feel better no matter what they do. That's right, one in three people will genuinely improve if you give them a nice, big glass of air instead of pink vovo berry juice. When we do research, we're trying to beat the placebo effect.

The best studies are large, double-blinded, randomized control trials. Say I take 5000 people. They're all wearing blindfolds. They're young, old, fat, thin men and women of various ethnicities, with multiple health care problems that are balanced out between both groups because we've got thousands of subjects.

A blind robot randomly hands half of them a glass of pink vovo berry juice and half of them a glass of flavoured water every morning. The robot checks how much pain they're in every day, if they can get back to work, if they don't need to take pain pills any more, if they can have sex (awfully nosy, those researchers, hmm?), or if they can now run marathons instead of still straining to tie their shoes at the end of six weeks.

This study is *large* (5000 people).

It's *double-blinded* because both the experimenter (the robot) and the subjects (the 5000 people) don't know if they're getting pink vovo berry juice or flavoured water.

It's *randomized*. Half the group is assigned to pink vovo berry juice, the other to water, and when you have such a big group, it tends to balance out the range in age, sex, ethnicity, medical problems, etc. in both groups.

That's the best kind of study. But it's expensive. And a lot of the time, nowadays, it's sponsored by the Vovojuju Corporation, which makes sure that the results come down hard on the side of pink vovo berry juice.

It also takes a lot of time and effort as well as money to get studies approved on human beings instead of on Petri dishes or on rats. Lots of times, things that look promising based on cells ("Neurons Bathed in Vovo Berry Extract Grow 20 Percent Longer!") or animal studies ("Paralyzed Dog Stands Up 24 Hours After Drinking Vovo Berry Juice!") just don't pan out on people.

So most studies are small. More like 30 people instead of 5000.

Many of them are not double-blinded. For example, acupuncture is impossible to double-blind. You can do sham acupuncture (applying needles to incorrect meridians) so that the patient is blinded ("I feel a needle. I just don't know if it's in the right place"), but whoever's putting the needles in either knows acupuncture or doesn't. So it's single instead of double-blinded. For double-blinding, you really would have to use a robot for the acupuncture, and that's…not in the cards yet.

So scientists do studies. Afterward, other researchers do a meta-analysis, or a study of the studies, pooling the evidence, deciding how good quality the research is. The Cochrane group in Australia is well-known for their meta-analyses, but other scientists do it, too.

We can end up grading all the research as level A, B, C and so on. Sometimes it's a bit of a grey area where the research goes, and of course it changes every time someone publishes a new study. But I promise I'll try and present it as fairly as possible.

*Pink vovo berry juice does not exist. No vovo berries were harmed in the writing of this book.

GRADE A WAYS TO FEEL BETTER

THE BED IS THE FRENEMY

Grade A recommendation: Don't get stuck in bed.[22] It's your frenemy (friend who's really the enemy)

I get it. You want to lie down, because moving hurts so much.

That can feel good for now. But in the long run, the bed is your enemy.

This is the one thing on back pain that we can all agree on. Grade A evidence.

You can recuperate a bit in bed, but you really want to try to get up, start moving, and get back to your normal life as soon as possible.

People who end up bedridden ultimately end up with more pain and a longer recovery.[23] A Finnish study found that bedridden patients had more pain, needed more time off work, and rated themselves as more disabled.[24]

Don't get stuck in bed unless you want to end up looking like Han Solo frozen in carbonite.

We used to tell people to rest in bed. Now we realize that you can end up with deconditioned muscles and worse off than you were before.

It's a crutch. You want to stop using it as soon as you can.

MOVING INTELLIGENTLY

Grade B recommendation: get back to your normal life.
I put it in the A section because if you don't want to get stuck in bed, we have to talk about how to get vertical.

I mentioned that quite often, a back pain patient will greet me standing up and say, "Sorry, I can't sit down."

To which I reply, "Great! Doesn't bother me if you want to stand up right now." In fact, I encourage it. I want my patients as pain-free as possible. So if your body is telling you to stand up, for the love of the big blue sky, *stand up.*

That's right. Your body is talking to you through pain.

Move this way, hurts a bit less.

Move that way, holy lickity split kitten burgers!

So listen to your body and move the way your body says to. It's in charge now. At least if you don't want to eat pain for the next few days.

Always **SCAN (slow-core-arms-nice)**.

Most people are afraid of making their pain worse, so they don't move. That's a normal fear, especially if you tried to keep working through it and now feel totally messed up. But studies show it's better to get back to usual routine and even work as much as you can, because it reduces pain and muscle spasm.

Listen to your body as you carefully ease yourself back into your normal activities, avoiding movements that hurt, like heavy lifting, prolonged sitting or standing, or twisting.

If you're not tuned into your body, you can consult someone who can give you a good overview. Are your muscles actually weak, or are the counter-muscles over-strengthened?

Do you need to work more on stretching or more on strengthening? Do you need to take a break between strengthening or work a little bit every day?

Don't be shy about asking for help, and if your advisor seems to be full of garbanzo beans, move on until you find someone who does work well with you, your body, your lifestyle, and your budget.

If your pain has a radicular component to it (sciatica pain that radiates down your leg), remember that the average patient like you takes longer to recover. So you may not want to jump back into the game right away. But the same rule still applies: move as much as your body allows, as soon and as intelligently as possible.

And always use common sense. I cheerfully reported to a friend that you can exercise through mild to moderate non-specific back pain, and she said, "Oh no. Do you think my husband should do that?" I told her, "Your husband has a burst fracture of his vertebra. That's not 'mild to moderate pain.' The bone is broken. He should follow whatever his surgeon and therapist told him."

However, most people can take every day slowly, focus on their bodies, and figure out what they need.

Of the billions of people in the world, you are the most familiar with your own body. If you can tune into it and figure out what you need, that's putting power into your own hands. This is all about you taking control of your own back.

DRUGS

Grade A recommendation: for <u>acute pain</u> <u>(<4-6 weeks)</u>, try acetaminophen, nonsteroidal anti-inflammatory drugs (NSAIDs), and possibly muscle relaxants.

Grade A to B recommendation: For <u>chronic pain</u> <u>(>6-12 weeks)</u>, try acetaminophen, NSAIDs, and maybe antidepressants, neuroleptics, or something like Tramadol.

You want fast relief? I've got to admit, drugs are the quickest route, but you've got to use medications sensibly.

There are three kinds of patients in the emergency room.

1) "Yeah, that's some shrapnel I got sticking out of my back for the past two years. I got it in Afghanistan. But I didn't want to take anything for it. I hate pills."

2) "I'm in so much pain! What the #@%$ is wrong with you? Give me everything you've got! I can't move! I'm dying here. AaaaaAAAAAAAaaaaaAAAAA! You're hurting me! I'm going to sue you! I'm allergic to NSAIDs! The only thing that works for me is Demerol! I hate this hospital! You're all a bunch of @#^@##@#%@#R@#F$%. Give me my Demerol NOW!"

3) I like the third kind of patient, the one in between these two extremes. Fortunately, this is the most common one. Here's Melissa's rule: **Drugs if necessary, but not necessarily drugs.**

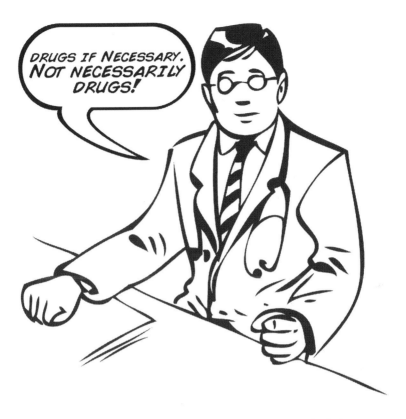

Look. Don't let your pain spiral out of control. If I ask you to rate your pain on a scale of 1 to 10—10/10 being someone ripping your leg, nose, and genitals off, and 1/10 almost unnoticeable— and you're truly at 20/10 (which a patient told me yesterday), that's no good. I'll have to work hard to get you down to 10/10 and then 8/10. And so forth.

But if you came in at 8/10, it takes fewer medications. I can get you home faster. Plus sitting in the waiting room won't be as excruciating.

On the other hand, if you come in trying to punch me in the face to make me give you IV morphine two seconds faster, news flash: not the best strategy.

Medications take the edge off. They make your pain bearable so you can get on with your construction company or your golf swing. But they're not the cure.

Sometimes people come back to the ER saying, "I still have pain."

Right. Because you're not cured. You're *palliated*. That means you feel better, but you haven't healed up. Maybe you're running at a 6/10, or 3/10, but you want zero pain.

That may not be in the cards. Your body has to heal itself. You may never get to zero. Most people do go down to a tolerable level, even to zero, within three to six weeks. And your chances are better than most if you're proactive. But in the meantime, use drugs only if necessary, because they can numb the pain while you take chances and aggravate your back all over again.

I'm not going to describe the strongest hospital medications, because you're not going to order them for yourself unless you're the face-puncher.

Don't be the face-puncher.

I envision medications like a pyramid. You start at the bottom of the pyramid and work your way up.

Of course I recommend that you chat with your friendly neighbourhood doctor before taking any medications (yep, even over-the-counter pills), to educate yourself, get a physical exam, and customize your treatment to your individual body instead of a one-size-fits-all meal deal. You should also bear in mind that research keeps changing, and you want the most up-to-date information.

1. Acetaminophen (Tylenol, Paracetamol)

The reason I suggest acetaminophen first-line is that it's relatively safe. So if it helps you, that's way cool, because it can save you from taking morphine and other narcotics, and healthy people can combine it with other medications.

However, I should mention that one randomized control study of 1652 people showed that acetaminophen wasn't any better than a placebo (fake) drug in getting people's pain down to zero or one out of ten.[25] So if it doesn't work for you, don't despair. Just keep climbing up the pyramid.

By the way, the same study found that it took 16 to 17 days for the average patient to get pain-free. So that's the kind of timeline we're looking at.

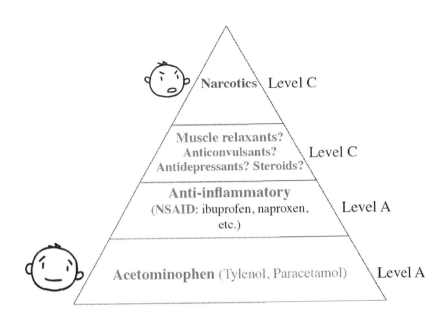

Worst case scenario, placebo drugs help about one third of people. So if you're one of about 30 percent who gets better on acetaminophen, hooray!

Dose: 325 mg to 1 gram (two 500 mg "extra strength") every six hours.

Do not take if you have: cirrhosis, other liver failure, overdosed on Tylenol already

Reduce dose if: you're over age 65

2. Anti-inflammatories (also called nonsteroidal anti-inflammatories, or NSAIDs)

NSAIDs work for back pain. They've been shown to work on both new and chronic (long-standing) pain, in a review of 65 different studies of over 11,000 people.[26]

Unless you have sciatica. Then their overall effect was no better than a placebo, so if you have pain shooting down your leg, you may have to keep moving up the pyramid, if you're not part of the lucky 30 percent that does get relief.

Also, bear in mind that anti-inflammatories can cause side effects, like ulcers or maybe even heart attacks, which is why they have the warning label about seeing a doctor.

For all NSAIDs, do not take if you have: kidney failure, heart disease, ulcers or other stomach problems. NSAIDs can make high blood pressure worse.

Reduce if: you're over age 65, have a sensitive stomach

2a) Ibuprofen (Advil, Motrin)

An anti-inflammatory. This is good. We want to get rid of inflammation. You can try the gel tablets to see if you absorb them more quickly.

Dose: 200 to 400 mg every six hours.

2b) Naproxen (Anaprox, Naprosyn)

Another anti-inflammatory. I like it because you only have to take it twice a day.

Dose: 250 to 500 mg every twelve hours.

There are other anti-inflammatories, but I'm not going to get into all of them. All NSAIDs work differently for different people. You may need to play around with your doctor/health care provider to find the correct one and the correct dose for you.

So what you're looking at is
1) Acetaminophen or NSAID
If that doesn't work, and your doctor gives you the thumbs up, you can add
2) Acetaminophen **plus** NSAID

If neither of these bring relief, we move up to the bigger guns that have more side effects—hence the unhappy face at the top of the pyramid.
3) Muscle relaxants
4) Anticonvulsants like topiramate
5) Antidepressants
6) Narcotics

MEDICATIONS WHERE YOU HAVE TO WEIGH THE PROS AND CONS:

3. Muscle relaxants (short term only)

Do they help? Some studies say yes, others say no. The big overall review in 2003 said that they could help, but should be used with caution.[27]

However, nurses and patients testify that these bad boys knock you out, and sometimes, what you need is a good night's sleep. Also, if patients tell me that muscle relaxants have helped before, it's a sign that they do respond to them. But these drugs are for acute, short-term pain, for only a week or two.

Do not use if you have kidney or liver disease, or glaucoma, or if you are elderly.

Can cause drowsiness, dizziness, dry mouth, and other side effects.

Do not drive.

Try to avoid carisoprodol (Soma) and diazepam (Valium) which are considered more addictive than the others.

4. Anticonvulsants

I know, I know. Why use anticonvulsant (epilepsy) drugs for back pain? Strangely enough, they might work.

At least one small but randomized control trial of topiramate (Topamax) in 96 patients showed it was better than placebo for chronic back pain,[28] and gabapentin (Neurontin) worked for chronic sciatica in an even smaller randomized control study (50 patients).[29]

Obviously, these drugs require more careful consideration. They're not the sort of thing we throw around like popcorn in the emergency department, but if you've got long-lasting pain or sciatica, they're an option.

5. Antidepressants

Your doctor might consider tricyclic antidepressants. One review showed they helped in patients with chronic pain, whether or not the patient was depressed.[30] Another meta-analysis concluded that it helped to reduce pain, but not to get people back in the saddle or other activities of daily living.[31]

In one randomized control trial, duloxetine (Cymbalta) reduced pain at 3 to 11 weeks, but at the end of the study (13 weeks), the effect had worn off.[32]

Personally, tricyclic antidepressants make me nervous because they're dangerous when you overdose on them. Again, these are for chronic pain and not my first choice in the emergency room.

6. Steroids

If you have back pain radiating down your leg, your doctor might suggest steroids, the big anti-inflammatory agents. There isn't any good research to back up spinal or trigger point injections, although we are trying to figure out if some patients are better candidates than others. More on that in the epidural steroids section.

Up until now, the studies on oral steroids (prednisone) haven't impressed, either. However, in a recent randomized control study of 269 patients with an acute, proven disc herniation on MRI, with mild to moderate disability from nerve pain radiating below the knee, two weeks of oral prednisone mildly reduced disability scores.[33]

It wasn't a cure-all. Scores tended to drop from severe disability to moderate at 3-4 weeks, hang out at moderate until 6 months, and finally regress to mild disability at a year. And no one wants even moderate pain for six months.

But in case it's an option for you, the study used a 15-day treatment course of prednisone: 60 mg for five days, then 40 mg per day for five days, ending with 20 mg per day for the last five days.

7. Narcotics (Opioids)

These are our biggest guns, so we only use them if we have to. Like, why use an AK-47 if a slingshot will get the job done?

Especially since, perhaps like an AK, narcotics can make you nauseous and confused. Or sleepy, delirious, constipated, and addicted.

If you've gotten on top of your pain, you're out of bed and getting back to your life, I hope you can bypass these bad boys.

If not, you and your doctor can work out a system. For example, just taking them at night so you can get that all-important good night's sleep.

However, bear in mind that one study showed 14 to 19 percent (that is, almost 1 in 5) people who'd never taken narcotics before, who got prescribed them for a painful condition, ended up coming back for another prescription.[34] That's a really high potential rate of addiction. And people who are *repeatedly* prescribed narcotics tend to do *worse*.

So this is a big question mark. Are you going to end up addicted?

Maybe.

Your doctor will decide whether or not to prescribe narcotics based on your history, physical exam, and possibly based on tests.

But if your doctor says no-go, he or she has a reason for it. Don't be a dink about it.

For all the following narcotics, here are the caveats.

Do not use if you're constipated. You'll have to add laxatives.

Do not drive.

Do not sell on the street.

Do not take them after the initial back pain. You can end up on them for the rest of your life. Many emergency departments have a non-renewal policy on narcotics, which means that you get one prescription, and after that, no luck.

Avoid if possible.

7a) Tramadol

In a study on chronic low back pain, tramadol worked better than placebo at reducing pain and getting people back to their activities of daily living.[35]

Dose: can start at 25 mg/day. In the study, the dose ranged from a total of 200 to 400 mg/day. Obviously, it's better if you have a doctor following you and adjusting the dose instead of just prescribing you a bunch of pills.

7b) Acetaminophen with codeine (Tylenol #3, Empracet)

Codeine doesn't work for 10 percent of Caucasians. So Tylenol #3 has a bad rap, that it doesn't work.

However, I like it because it's less likely to make you high and therefore has little street value. It also works in 90 percent of white people, which is a pretty good rate. (By the way, lots of blood pressure medications have high failure rates in black people, because fewer studies are done on people of colour, but we prescribe them to black people anyway and shrug our shoulders when they don't work. Just saying.)

Most of my patients are indeed Caucasian. I just ask them, "Have you ever used Tylenol #3? Does it work for you?" If the answer is yes, I consider prescribing it.

Dose: 325 mg with 30 mg of codeine, one to two tablets every six hours

6c) Acetaminophen with Oxycodone (Percocet)

This one works in most people. It also makes you high. That's why we try not to prescribe it. It does have street value. It's more addictive. Little old ladies are terrified of it. But if you have a lot of pain, your doctor may consider prescribing it for you.

Dose 1/2 or 1-2 tablets every 6 hours.

Remember, drugs only if necessary. That's my last paranoid reminder that narcotics (Tramadol, Tylenol #3, and Percocet) and the other C drugs have lots of side effects and you should stop them as soon as you can.

Basically, we're still figuring out how to deal with nerve pain, the kind of pain that runs down your legs. So far, we don't have any easy answers. Acetaminophen and NSAIDs don't work as well for nerve pain, so you'll have to try other medications *or* step up your game in trying everything else in an attempt to decrease your need for medication.

Pain is a warning sign. It's like you're driving your car and your dashboard light is flashing. You can keep driving, and sometimes everything turns out okay. But if you need a tire patched to get to the garage, medication is the tire patch.

So if you need drugs, just accept this temporary gift of drugs.

But once you get to the garage, try and figure out what's under the hood and what's causing the pain so you can wean yourself off the drugs as soon as you can.

It is easier to find men who will volunteer to die,
than to find those who are willing to endure pain with patience.
—Julius Caesar

DON'T I NEED AN MRI?

If you have red flags, you need urgent imaging.
Otherwise, most people can avoid imaging for the first month or two (Grade A[36] **recommendation for chronic pain and Grade C recommendation**[37] [38] **for acute pain.)**

Everyone knows X-rays. You've also probably heard of advanced imaging techniques like magnetic resonance imaging (MRIs) or computerized tomography (CT or CAT scans). Shouldn't you have them early and often?

Actually, earlier imaging studies don't make you feel any better. They don't help you heal faster. They do cost cash and make it more likely that you'll end up on a surgeon's table, if you're into that.

The problem is that most adults have some sort of crap in their backs. You take a picture of it, you see it and say, "Aha! That's it! That's my pain!" But actually, that's usually not the answer. The picture's abnormality may not correspond to the area where you have pain. And lots of people who have no pain would have the same (or worse) scans.

The evidence: a 2009 mega-review of acute and subacute back pain, comparing over a thousand people's combined outcomes at 3, 6, and 12 months if they had imaging or not. No difference.[39]

Well, what if you're a senior? Another study looked at people aged 65 or over, without leg symptoms, who got imaging within 6 weeks or not. No difference.[40] (It's not a coincidence that they excluded people with sciatica, a condition which is more complicated and needs more individual attention.)

So who *does* need imaging?

The red flag people. That's less than one percent of people coming to see a regular doctor.

But in case that's you, a reminder to keep an eye out for these symptoms and signs:

1. *Neurological*: it's bad news if you can't handle your pee or poop, can't feel the toilet paper when you wipe, and/or have a worrisomely weak limb ("It hurts too much to move, Doc" doesn't count, so let your doctor assess this one).

2. *Fever, chills, and tenderness in your spine that suggests an abscess:* lemme load you in the machine and take a good look.

3. *Cancer.* I'm not going to joke about this one. No one likes cancer.

All I'm saying is, yes, you hurt, and no, you probably don't need to spend the next 45 minutes in an MRI. It may also not be worth the radiation risk of a CT scan or even the more minor radiation from an X-ray.

This is a judgment call. Let your health care provider explain why you do or don't need the scan.

Another tip: if you get pulled into the emergency department immediately, and are surrounded by doctors and nurses wearing face masks, inserting lines in you, and asking you if you want a priest, this is not good.

Don't envy the people pulled ahead of you. It's usually a bad sign.

ACUPUNCTURE

Grade A recommendation: try acupuncture for chronic pain

Cool fact: we may have been using acupuncture to treat back pain for the past 5000 years.

Have you heard of the "Tyrolean ice man"? They found that poor guy in 1991, frozen in the Alps for the past five millennia. His skeleton showed signs of significant back arthritis. The tattoos inside his heels and Achilles tendons correspond exactly to Chinese acupressure points.

Current studies show that acupuncture can help chronic back pain today.

Acupuncture's effects seemed to be comparable to conventional medicine and injectable anti-inflammatories in a small but randomized study of severely disabled patients.[41] So if you'd rather get acupuncture needles than Western doctor needles, that's a good thing. And if you say, no way, gimme a shot, regular doc, it's all good too.

In a study comparing acupuncture and massage, where participants got to choose between them, acupuncture did help, but the effect was more pronounced for the people who chose acupuncture.[42]

Acupuncture studies tend to be small, and it's hard to blind participants because they can tell if they're getting needles in their skin or not. As I mentioned, the studies try to blind participants by having the practitioner insert needles into areas that are not on the correct meridian for the pain. They also tend to study acupuncture in patients who have chronic pain instead of acute pain.

However, a meta-analysis of 29 randomized control trials including nearly 18,000 patients analyzed the results for back, shoulder, and neck pain and concluded that acupuncture seemed to help more than placebo. Interestingly, even sticking needles in incorrect meridians seemed to help, but the authors thought real acupuncture had a benefit on top of that.[43]

A joint statement from the American College of Physicians and the American Pain Society gave acupuncture the thumbs up in 2007 for people with chronic pain who didn't respond to other treatments.[44] The North American Spine Society said it helps with short-term pain compared to doing nothing, and you can do both acupuncture and traditional Western medicine in combo.[45] Plus a good review article gave acupuncture an A rating for chronic back pain[46].

I wouldn't be a doctor if I didn't caution you about some of the drawbacks, including skin irritation or infection, hematoma (bleeding), the needles becoming dislodged or moving to different spots, and pneumothorax (needle in the lung)[47].

TL;DR: if your back pain has been dragging on for six weeks or more, and you're not needle-phobic, you might want to give acupuncture a try.

GRADE B WAYS TO FEEL BETTER

EXERCISE AND EDUCATION

Grade B recommendation: exercise and educate yourself to prevent back pain for up to a year.

So what helps prevent low back pain from smacking you in the spine?

Exercise plus education about back pain.

That's the conclusion from the 2016 meta-analysis by Dr. Daniel Steffens and colleagues at the University of Sydney, looking at 21 randomized control trials of 30,850 people.[48]

Exercise plus education reduces your risk of a back pain episode by 25 to 40 percent (moderate-quality evidence).

I'm excited about this. The fact that you're reading this book means you want to educate yourself. I just hope you want to move your bum as well.

Exercise and education are our secret weapon. I'm going to call it **E2**. (You have to a have a cute name for things. My kids and I left *Star Wars: The Force Awakens* movie squealing about robot BB-8.)

Exercise alone might help reduce your risk by 35 percent and your need for sick leave by 78 percent, although those studies were considered low- to very low-quality evidence.

Education without exercise didn't show an effect (low- and very low-quality evidence again). You gotta move.

Effects died off after a year. No surprise there. Keep moving and keep your brain ticking.

Most studies didn't show a clear win for exercising right away for acute, short term pain. But you can start educating yourself immediately and get back to your normal routine as you're able. If you're already an athlete or otherwise attuned to your body, that'll be sooner rather than later.

As soon as your body allows it, and if you've been hauling this back pain around for over six weeks, ease yourself into an exercise routine, baby. Exercise will improve your function and get you back to work.[49]

The **E2** study was a meta-analysis, so they included a whole hodge podge of exercise programs from multiple studies, as long as the study was well-built.

"There was some variation, but in general, trials included exercises to improve strength, flexibility, skill and aerobic fitness," said Steffens in an interview. "The exercises did not just focus on the spine but included upper and lower limb exercises as well."

Workout frequency varied too, but study participants would exercise in the clinic two or three times a week, plus additional exercises at home, for eight weeks to 18 months.

The good news is, **E2** becomes a Choose Your Own Pain-Free Back Adventure. You can customize your own program to whatever type of exercise you enjoy doing, because when they look at the results overall, you cut your chance of a back blowout by a third, for up to a year. As long as you keep exercising.

If you're an athlete, you probably know what to do already.

If you have no clue, I suggest start off with walking. It's free and you know how to do it. If you want to step it up to running, swimming, yoga, salsa, or biking, you will eventually discover activities you enjoy and honestly want to incorporate into your life.

"If there were a pill out there that could reduce your risk of future episodes of back pain by 30 percent, I'd probably be seeing ads on television every night," said Dr. Tim Carey, who co-wrote a commentary on the article.[50]

TL;DR: Exercise and educate yourself (E2). If you had to pick only one of the two, exercise. But if you do both, your chances of developing a random lower back pain blowout are cut by a third.

If you're ready now, jump to the E2 section.

AEROBIC EXERCISE

WALKING

Walk to reduce your back pain (Grade B or C evidence).

For chronic pain, there's fair evidence that walking helps reduce pain for up to eight weeks after the injury. After that, walking doesn't so much reduce pain as help you get back to your normal activities, but the effects last even longer, up to a year.[51]

Strangely enough, there aren't that many studies on walking and back pain. A 2010 review just didn't show enough data on it to draw any conclusions.[52]

Maybe it's too simple, or there aren't any corporations that have patented it yet. But I feel pretty confident recommending good, old-fashioned putting one foot in front of the other.

SWIMMING AND AQUA FITNESS

Grade B or C evidence: If you like swimming or other aqua-based activities, try them.

Water makes you buoyant. You're floating instead of bouncing on your joints. The water sweeps your sweat away. You might feel more relaxed than if you were pounding on pavement.

It's a total body workout. Instead of worrying which move is for your back, core, glutes, arms, legs, or heart, good news—it's for everything! Burn calories, lose weight, get flexible, do resistance training against the water, have fun.

Don't know how to swim?

Walk into the pool until the water reaches your chest height and start walking in place. That's how a therapist might start you off anyway.

There are also pool aerobics programs and...swimming lessons!

An aqua fitness group five times a week could decrease your pain, improve your mood, and cut your fat-to-muscle ratio. That's what a small randomized control trial found.[53] A review said that most studies gave water the thumbs up but were not good quality.[54] Another review concluded that aqua-based therapy might not be better than any other kind of conservative treatment.

Again, even if there's not a ton of studies behind them, we say water-based exercise is good for you.

Two caveats: you might want to get the thumbs up from your doctor before you start a new exercise program, and you might have to start slow. Five minutes of water walking is cool beans for a beginner.

YOGA

Grade B evidence: If you've always wanted to try yoga, now is the time to take the first step. Or breath. Or posture.

We have evidence that yoga helps back pain, especially if you're open to the idea[55]: at least one paper says there's strong evidence that yoga helps reduce pain and functional disability in the short term and moderate evidence that it helps in the long term, too.[56]

Yoga can seem intimidating because the media likes to show pictures of people (mostly skinny Indian guys or beaming, fresh-faced women) pretzeling themselves. So yes, if you're a newbie, you want to be careful choosing a type of yoga and a teacher open to beginners.

One large, randomized control trial focused on Viniyoga, which reduced pain and "bothersomeness" scores more than traditional exercise programs plus a self-care booklet. The Viniyogis also needed fewer pain medications.[57]

So Viniyoga, with gentle postures flowing from one to the next, as well as breathing and chanting, is a good choice to start out.

Iyengar yoga pays a lot of attention to alignment and uses props, so even if you're stiff, they'll figure out how to adapt to you.

Hatha yoga is a broad term that generally means you'll be moving during class. It's more physical than meditative. That's the kind I do. I just like to move.

These three types of yoga reduced pain and disability scores in two different reviews, one by Posadzki and Ernst[58] and one by Cramer and company.[59] A meta-analysis by Chou and Huffman[60] found the level of evidence wasn't so hot and gave the thumbs up to Viniyoga, but judged two studies on Iyengar yoga as inconclusive.

Another review by McCall et al thought yoga was unlikely to harm you, and that depression, anxiety, and various pain disorders might be helped by both Hatha yoga and restorative (therapeutic, using props to adapt to students' bodies) yoga.[61]

If you're already an athlete, you might like to try more challenging styles, like Vinyasa, Ashtanga, or Bikram, although these haven't been analyzed for effectiveness in preventing and treating back pain.

Personally, I love yoga. If I do some mild yoga exercises, in anywhere from five minutes to forty minutes, depending how bad the pain is, I can go from gritted teeth, hunched over and hobbling, to my husband saying, "Hey, you don't look so bad now." He's an engineer, better at observing computer systems than people, but he can see that I'm standing more upright. I also feel more calm and kind-hearted after yoga.

Lots of studios will let you try your first class free, or at a serious discount. You can also look at YouTube videos, but if you don't know what you're doing, a teacher can really accelerate your learning and make sure you don't hurt yourself.

Don't be afraid to ask your teachers questions about their training and experience. They may belong to the Yoga Alliance or the International Association of Yoga Therapists.

Feel free to try different studios and different teachers until you find the right fit. Once you're comfortable, you can practice at home or in a studio; the McCall study didn't show a difference between them.

PILATES

Pilates can help, too. A meta-analysis concluded, based on some low-quality studies, that Pilates is probably better than doing nothing to reduce pain and disability, in the short term and intermediate term.[62]

I know, it sounds like a lukewarm recommendation, doesn't it? But Pilates is big into strengthening your core, and you know I'm down with that. Plus, who wouldn't want less pain or disability?

There's no proof it's better than any other type of exercise, but if Pilates is your thang, get your thang on.

PHYSIOTHERAPY AND SPINE STABILIZATION EXERCISES

If you're in a new bout of pain, physiotherapy and spine stabilization exercises may decrease both your need to visit the doctor and the chance of another back pain episode (Grade B evidence).

Lots of physiotherapists recommend the McKenzie exercises designed for sciatic-type pain, which you can view on YouTube here: http://bit.ly/1pQSTuB

For acute back pain, McKenzie exercises appeared to help slightly, but have not been scientifically proven to be more effective than any other low back treatments.[63] [64]As I discuss in the sciatica section, McKenzie exercises may be better reserved for patients with bulging discs.

Long-term, physio seems to decrease need for health care services,[65] which I consider a win; who wants to sit around in a waiting room all the time?

For chronic back pain, it may help a little for pain in the short term.[66]

Sometimes physiotherapists offer modalities like TENS and ultrasound. These treatments have *not* been shown to reduce back pain (I cover them under grade C evidence), so I encourage you to get hands-on exercise instruction from the physio. You're better off exercising at home or better yet, outdoors, instead of paying for unproven toys.

CHIROPRACTORS

In plain English: **if you just hurt your back in the last month or two, a chiropractor can make you feel better, but the effects don't last long term.**

There's level B evidence that chiropractors are no better than sticking to regular doctors and NSAIDs for acute pain.[67]

Spinal manipulative therapy by chiropractors, osteopaths, and other therapists appears "no better and no worse" than other treatments for chronic, non-specific low back pain that has lasted 12 weeks or more.[66]

Short term, for acute and subacute low back pain patients, chiropractors may reduce pain and disability. Medium term, they can help with pain. But they have no proven long term benefits (like at the one to two year mark), and no significant effect on chronic pain. Most chiropractor studies are biased.[68]

People like chiropractors. One study compared patients who received a chiropractic treatment vs. seeing a physiotherapist vs. getting a booklet on exercises to do at home. People with a booklet improved as much as with a physiotherapist or a chiropractor, which emphasizes my two main points—your body wants to heal itself, and you've got to exercise—but they were happier with a physiotherapist or chiropractor (75 percent satisfied) than with only the pamphlet (30 percent).[69] Of course it feels nicer to sit down with someone instead of getting a piece of paper and a metaphorical boot in the rear end, but in the end, the physio/chiro/booklet groups had similar disability claims, need for bed rest, and recurrent back pain.

If you've got extra money and insurance coverage, or you enjoy spinal manipulation, you can book an appointment.

However, I *never* advise high-velocity chiropractic neck manipulation because of the risk of stroke[70] and even death.[71]

MULTIDISCIPLINARY REHABILITATION

What if you got a whole team on your side? A physician plus at least one other worker from another area like psychology, social work, or occupational health?

If you can get into a program like that, some studies show that you'll feel less pain, report less disability, get back to work five weeks earlier, and need a week less of sick time in your first year. This kind of improvement can last up to five years![72]

Obviously, programs like this are expensive and aren't standardized. Another study showed "disappointing" results.[73] But if my work place offered it to me for free, I'd give it a try. And if I could get into the one that resulted in five years of relief, I'd sign up immediately.

YELLOW FLAGS

Usually, people feel sideswiped by back pain and betrayed by their bodies. But the real mystery is, why do some people end up completely borked by back pain and others take a lickin' and keep on tickin', even though their MRI studies look the same?

It's a delicate subject, but it circles back to the question, *Is something else going on in your life?*

Dr. Jack Stern talks about an eminent doctor with excruciating back pain who was also trying to take care of his invalid wife. The doctor was afraid he'd end up in a wheelchair like his own father.[74] No one had ever talked to him about what was going on in his life. He was such a well-known doctor, they didn't want to offend him or intrude. But actually, it just left him isolated and in pain. That doctor ended up taking stock of his own life and deciding to retire so he could move to a warmer climate and focus on taking care of his wife and himself instead of knocking himself out at the university. Your mileage may vary, but it just goes to show, this isn't just a problem for people on disability programs. Problems beget more problems.

This isn't something we talk about in the emergency department, but maybe we should. There's **level B evidence that you're at higher risk of getting chronic pain if you have "yellow flags"** like

Mood problems: often anxiety or depression

Work: sorry to say, if you have a worker's compensation claim or legal action going on, you're more likely to be disabled. Also, hands up if you hate your job.

Social: you have a history of abuse or your family is over-protective.

Age: you're older

Behaviour: you can't cope, you can't sleep, you stop activities and feel indifferent about treatment

Take an honest look at yourself, and if any of these things are an issue for you, I salute you if you can talk to your health care provider and/or someone else you trust.

You are not just your back. You're a whole person, and we have to think about how all of you is dealing with the situation, not just your skeletal muscle cells. If this makes sense to you, you can jump to the section called Getting Your Heart on Your Side.

COGNITIVE BEHAVIOUR THERAPY AND RELAXATION

Grade B evidence: cognitive behavioural therapy and progressive relaxation can help your chronic back pain [75] in the short-term (moderate-quality evidence).[76]

You may have heard of cognitive behavioural therapy (CBT) because it was originally developed to retool thinking patterns in depression, but now CBT is used in a variety of conditions.

A Cochrane meta-analysis reviewed 30 different studies of chronic low back pain with a total of 3438 participants. CBT can be divided into three different schools

1) operant: works on the external factors associated with your pain;

2) cognitive: focuses on your feelings, thoughts, and/or beliefs about the pain);

3) respondent (biofeedback on your muscle activity. When your muscles get tense, you learn how to relax them).

First, the most impressive news. Cochrane decided there was moderate-quality evidence that behavioural therapy was *better* than usual care (which consisted of mostly physical therapy, medical treatments, and/or back school, depending on the study) for pain relief in the short term. However, intermediate or long term, the effect wore off. There was no difference in function. And strangely enough, for people whose back pain was so bad, they had to get admitted to hospital, adding behavioural therapy to their regular rehabilitation made no difference.

Intermediate or long term, behaviour therapy got pretty much the same results as...wait for it...exercise.

Operant or cognitive or combination CBT were pretty much the same, in terms of short term pain relief. And operant therapy reduced short-term pain more than hanging out on a waiting list. How's that for a sterling recommendation?

TL;DR: CBT can help reduce chronic back pain in the short term, but in the end, exercise is just as good.

GRADE C WAYS TO FEEL BETTER

HOT OR COLD?

Short version: maybe apply heat for the first five days or up to two weeks. [77]

I've heard doctors go hard core on this. "Ice! Only ice your back! Heat is the devil!" Others say, "You must alternate or reap the consequences!" Well, they make not quite invoke Satan, but that's the idea.

I say, "What makes your body feel better?" That's the cardinal rule here.

Neither heat nor cold have been proven to speed up healing over the long term, but heat wrap therapy showed a small win.[78] Both of them can alleviate pain in the short term.[79] Two thumbs up for pain relief.

Heat increases inflammation, which relaxes muscles and might help heal.

Now, wait a minute. Didn't I tell you to take anti-inflammatories (NSAIDs) if you can tolerate them? Yes, I did. Inflammation causes pain and swelling. But that's really how the body repairs itself. If an area is inflamed, the body sends out chemical signals saying "This is the bad zone!" and then cells come to repair it.

Maybe think of inflammation like road construction and repair in the summer. If it gets out of hand, it's a nightmare. But it's also a necessary step to keep our roads running.

The Cochrane review showed that heat wraps can help a little bit.

So if heat makes your body feel better, go for it.

If you like heat, you can try a bath or shower, or the bean bag in the microwave.

I suggest four times a day, 15 minutes at a time.

Ice is nice because 1) It numbs the area, which directly reduces the ouchies.

2) It makes the area less inflamed because blood vessels shrink. The muscles in the vessel walls constrict when it's cold. Don't worry, they'll open up again when it's warmer out. It's like Canadians flying to Florida when it's cold and coming back for the summer.

3) We do know that nerve conduction speeds up with cold. At least one neurosurgeon[80] theorizes this can reduce muscle spasm.

On the other hand, a big review study of ice vs. heat didn't show that ice reduced pain and disability. But if it helps you, why not?

Wrap the ice in a towel so that it's not unpleasant, or use one of those bean bags you can stick in the freezer (or fridge, if the freezer is too intense). Some people like to use frozen peas and let the cold bag mold to the injury, which is fine if you don't mind wasting food.

I recommend four times a day, 15 minutes at a time.

If you can't do it that often, try to do it as often as you can.

Once your back doesn't hurt as much, you'll naturally spend less time icing or heating your back, which is fine.

HERBAL REMEDIES

Grade B or C evidence: Cayenne *(Capsicum frutescens)*, devil's claw, or white willow bark might be more effective than placebo for chronic pain. [81]

About half our medications are derived from plants. Here are the top three herbal contenders, all based on the same meta-analysis.[82]

1. Cayenne pepper derivative may be better than placebo, based on low to very low quality evidence. So once in a while, I prescribe capsicum cream to chronic low back patients who feel like they've tried everything else, with a warning not to touch their eyes, nose, mouth or genitals afterward. 'Cause that's not the kind of genital burning most of us are looking for.

2. *Salix alba* (white willow bark). This is where aspirin comes from, so maybe it's not surprising that 120 mg or 240 mg salicin every day can help bring down pain in the short term and decrease the need for other medications (moderate quality evidence). One study also showed a "minimal" effect on platelet function, though, also like aspirin, so be careful if you're at risk for bleeding.

3. I admit it sounds pretty wild to take devil's claw *(Harpagophytum procumbens)*, but 50 mg or 100 mg of harpagoside may be better than placebo in terms of reducing pain and the need for rescue medication (low quality evidence).

Herbal runners-up include a study of Brazilian arnica *(Solidago chilensis M)* with only 20 patients that was considered very low-quality evidence, and comfrey root extract *(Symphytum officinale L)*, which was also rated as low-quality evidence.

Always look for standardized dosing for herbal remedies, because they're not held to the same pharmacological standard as regular medication. You could end up paying big bucks for a bottle of nothing.

TL;DR: If you have chronic pain and you like herbs, try cayenne *(Capsicum frutescens)*, white willow bark, or devil's claw.

EPIDURAL STEROID INJECTIONS

Grade B and C recommendation: epidural steroids *won't* help you in the long term. Trigger point injections don't help, either.

Epidural steroid injections mean a needle into your back, just outside the spinal cord, with a strong anti-inflammatory medication (steroids). You've probably heard of epidurals for women in labour. This is the same idea, only with steroids instead of, or in addition to, pain medications.

It's something we try when we don't have a lot of options. You're in pain, usually chronic pain, without relief. Someone says, "Why don't I put a needle in your back? That might help."

Trigger point injections means injecting steroids, anaesthetics, or saline into trigger points, which are spots of irritated muscle.

Studies haven't shown any clear evidence over placebo for either type of injection.

There's such poor proof for steroid injections that, as I said above, it's a grade B recommendation that you *don't* get epidural injections. You should also consider the risks of unusual complications like bleeding, nerve damage, or epidural abscesses, as well as a small amount of radiation exposure.

But of course some people feel better after getting a steroid injection. Which makes you wonder if it's the placebo effect, or if we're doing it wrong. For example, one theory is that a biomarker like the fibronectin aggrecan complex can predict who's going to respond to an epidural injection.[83] Another theory is that we should use ultrasound to find trigger points instead of basing the injection on the physical exam.[84] Plus, different doctors inject different substances and different locations, so it's hard to do a meta-analysis.

Regardless, at this point, there's no proof that epidural and trigger point injections help more than a placebo. On the other hand, they didn't rule out that it could help some people, if we could figure out who those people were. [85]

We do know a few things:

1. Epidural steroids should be saved for people who have pain for over six weeks,[86] *and*

2. For those who have radicular symptoms (pain going down the leg).[87]

They don't help at all if you have advanced spinal stenosis[88] or stenosis of more than three lumbar vertebrae.[89]

TL;DR: No proof that it works. Your doctor might suggest it if you've had sciatica for more than 6 weeks, but it does carry risks.

PROLOTHERAPY

Grade C evidence: Prolotherapy alone is *not* an effective treatment for back pain[90]

Prolotherapy means injecting things like dextrose (a sugar) or lidocaine (an anaesthetic) into ligaments, based on the theory that this will strengthen the ligament.

Don't expect prolotherapy to help your back pain on its own, based on a Cochrane meta-analysis of five studies. The two studies of prolotherapy alone did not help.

The other three studies combined prolotherapy with exercise, spinal manipulation, and other treatments, and did show a benefit, but the problem is, you don't know what's helping—the prolotherapy, the exercise, the spinal manipulation, the phase of the moon, etc.

In medical school, I was taught not to inject a ligament more than three times, for fear of weakening the ligament. Not everyone adheres to this rule, but keep caution in mind, especially if you don't know what substance they're injecting into you and what benefit you'll get from it.

ULTRASOUND

Grade C evidence: "We did not find any convincing evidence that ultrasound is an effective treatment for low back pain." [91]

That was the conclusion by the Cochrane meta-analysis of randomized control trials of 362 adults with chronic, non-specific (no precise diagnosis) back pain.

Sounds pretty damning, but I have to say that of the extra modalities offered by physiotherapists, there is at least moderate-quality evidence that it might help low back function in chronic patients in the short term. The effect is so small that many people won't see the difference, but I'll just point out that almost everything else in the Grade C section is focusing on low- and very low-quality evidence of slight differences in pain.

So right now, there's no good evidence for ultrasound. However, if you like to spend money, it's better than TENS or Low Level Laser Therapy.

TENS

Transcutaneous Electrical Nerve Stimulation (TENS) is no better than placebo and does not help you get back to your normal activities.[92] [93] [94] [95] [96]
(Grade B evidence that this is *not* worthwhile)

TENS sounds nice and possibly scientific: someone puts electrodes on your skin, and the current stimulates peripheral nerves, which is supposed to stop pain signals. But a meta-analysis of four high quality randomized controlled trials showed the same results as placebo.

Not recommended, unless you like the buzz.

LOW LEVEL LASER THERAPY

Grade C evidence: not enough data to recommend Low Level Laser Therapy [97]

The theory behind Low Level Laser Therapy (LLLT), sometimes called biostimulation or photobiology, is that applying single-wavelength light treatment helps repair connective tissue and reduce inflammation.

The studies are all small, using different populations and different wavelengths of light. Out of seven studies, three showed a small reduction in pain in the first three to six months, but the results were not impressive, and the study sizes and designs were so variable that the Cochrane meta-analysis basically said, "Can't say anything for sure based on these crappy studies. Do some good randomized control trials."

MASSAGE

Grade C evidence: Massage may reduce pain, but only in the short term (low-quality and very low-quality evidence).[98]

Mmmm, massage. Would that help your back?

Cherkin et al's study found that maybe massage could bring down your pain about 2/10 points on the 10 point scale in the short term, but after six months or a year, massage made no difference.[99]

Study participants who didn't get massages improve over time as well, 1/10 points on the 10 point scale, so you can see the pain difference is very small.

The good news is, it doesn't seem to matter what kind of massage you get. "Relaxation" or "advanced" massage got the same results. So you don't have to pay extra for anyone with fancy-sounding credentials.

Also, unlike acupuncture, you don't have to worry about a punctured lung as an (unlikely) side effect. The main drawbacks were a) the cost and b) the fact that 1.5 to 25 percent of people complained of increased pain afterward.[100] So if your therapist is too vigorous, you can ask him or her to back off.

Most studies selected chronic pain patients, although one focused on people with acute back pain.

Thus, evidence points toward exercising your own body instead of having someone else rub your naked flesh. Awwww.

BACK BRACES

Grade C evidence: Back braces, corsets, etc. don't prevent back pain.[101]

You can wear them if you want, but the concern is that you'd be better off developing your core, which is a natural brace, instead of relying on an external belt. So if it helps to wear them for a few days, okay, but also start exercising.

And make sure that you know how lift properly without needing a brace.

PROPER LIFTING

Preparation: assess the object to make sure it's not too heavy, that it's packed properly and won't shift while you're carrying it, and that you can get a good grip.

Face the object—don't twist to the side.

Activate the core muscles.

Keep your back straight, not hunched.[102]

Keep the load close to your body, not at arms' length, and around chest level[103] (between shoulders and waist). Think Goldilocks here: not too high, not too low, not at arms' length. Juuuuuust right.

I've had a few patients come in with back pain after they were carrying a heavy load with someone who dropped the other end. You can't control that, so I guess the only thing I would say is, be aware that your partner may flake out, and if you can work out a plan B, like a fork lift, so much the better.

POSTURE

I've been slouching since I was eleven years old. My mom always told me to stand up straight. Would that prevent back pain?

Not so much. A 2008 review of studies to date couldn't prove that the curve of your back caused back pain.[104] The investigators measured not only spinal curves, but leg length and muscle length on 600 people, and none definitively caused back pain.[105]

However, I have to admit that I try not to slump because it looks lame, and bad posture won't help back pain, either. So here are a few quick tips in a "do as I say, not as I do" sort of way, starting from the bottom up.

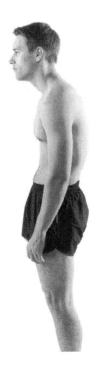 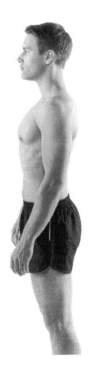

FEET

Try to balance your weight between your feet.

One way to check is to step on two different weight scales at once, putting one foot on each. I did this exercise at the mall and the guy was like, "Try to balance both sides."

I said, "I am."

"You have a ten-pound difference between your feet."

"Oh." I didn't think much about it until a decade later, when my acupuncture doctor remarked that I shift all my weight to my right foot, the "yang" side, the "male," outward-energy, ambition side. That's even with yoga trying to rebalance me. Yikes.

So don't be me. Try and place equal weight on each foot.

PELVIS

Pelvis: aim it back, like you've got a tail, instead of tucking it under like a scolded dog.

But don't stick it out too far. You'll end up swaybacked.

BACK

Check your rear view in the mirror. See how there's a vertical indentation for the spine? The muscles on either side of your spine should look equal instead of one side jutting out.

CORE

These are the muscles around your midsection. I go into this in more detail in the anatomy section, but I find that if I maintain some tension in my core, like a belt ("the abdominal draw-in maneuver"), my posture automatically improves. It makes me look thinner, too.

And that's an easy way to keep your front ribs aligned with your pelvis, instead of over-arching your back again. You don't want the banana back.

Plus, I've heard that if you keep the core engaged, that's the best core exercise of all. Not miserable crunching and endless plank poses, but mindfully using your core every waking minute. I couldn't find a study to back it up, although this one examined muscle size under ultrasound.[106] Worth a try, right?

SHOULDERS

Who carries tension in their shoulders and back? Hands up!
Or rather, don't keep those hands and shoulders lifted up.
Try to keep your shoulders down and relaxed if you notice that they tend to gravitate toward your ears.

HEAD

Keep your head balanced in line with your spine. Look at the horizon, which will automatically straighten out your shoulders.

I know it sounds like a lot of things to worry about at once.

QUICK TIP: BALANCE A BOOK ON YOUR HEAD.

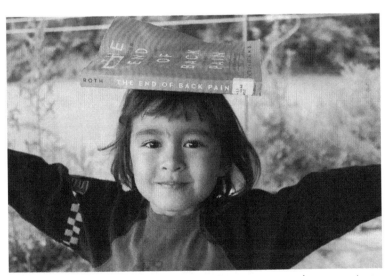

It's hard to remember all of these factors, so a short cut is to balance a book on top of your head.

True, you will look odd. But instinctively, as soon as you try walking or sitting with a paperback resting on your crown, you will adopt a more adaptive posture. It's a reminder to keep your shoulders back and even and your pelvis out but not too far out. I'm writing this right now with a book on my head. Try it!

You don't have to work like this all the time (although I'd like to see this start as a trend), but it gets you into the right habit. And that's all you need.

If you want to spend more time on your posture, Esther Gokhale's book, *8 Steps to a Pain-Free Back*,[107] has a lot of cross-cultural pictures illustrating the "right" and "wrong" way to stand, sit, or walk. I was also stunned to see a picture of someone sitting on a stool in an operating room with his arms crossed and shoulders slumped while he stared at the OR tables. That was like me!

TL;DR: correcting your posture hasn't been proven to help your back pain, but it can't hurt. Walk around with a book on your head to look extra-cool.

SLEEP

"Pain and sleep are integrally connected."
—David Neumeyer, MD, Associate Director of the Sleep
Disorder Center at the Lahey Clinic Medical Center[108]

Pain wakes you up. Sixty-five percent of people with chronic pain wake up in the middle of the night because of, you guessed it, pain.[109] So back pain causes insomnia.

But as neurologist Charles Bae points out, "On the flip side, sleep deprivation can lower your pain threshold and pain tolerance and make existing pain feel worse."

So you end up in this vicious circle/chicken-and-egg deal. You can't sleep because you have pain and you have more pain because you can't sleep. WTH?

You need to cut this sucker off and sleep. But how?

Well, if you're at the point where drugs are necessary, you can use drugs to cut the pain.

And you can consider a change in your mattress and in your sleep position.

THE BEST MATTRESS

Q. What kind of mattress should I buy?
A. What kind of mattress does your body like?

The party line is to recommend hard mattresses, but it really depends on what works for your body. One study of chronic back pain patients compared medium-hard mattresses to hard mattresses, and the medium-hard group had less pain.[110]

So try out different mattresses. Roll around on them. If you've got a partner, pile in, because more bodies will change the firmness.

You can also try sleeping on the floor, on a tatami mat. See what your body likes.

LIDOCAINE PATCHES AND OTHER TOPICALS

Lidocaine is a topical anaesthetic. You can get a patch, cream, spray, or plaster. It numbs the skin. There's some very low-quality evidence that it might help nerve pain, but nothing proven,[111] and nothing specific for back pain. We're waiting for some bigger studies going on right now.

Tiger Balm and other skin creams may make your skin tingle, but they don't penetrate below the skin. Use 'em only if you like 'em.[112]

ESSENTIAL OILS

Grade C: Not enough evidence to recommend lavender or other essential oils

I found a gazillion websites touting essential oils, but only one randomized control trial testing them: eight weeks of acupressure with lavender oil seemed to improve pain and mobility.[113] That's only one small study of 61 patients, and you have to ask if it was the acupressure, the lavender oil, or both (assessed as very low-quality evidence). We already know that acupuncture is better than placebo. Acupressure means the practitioners rubs you with their hands instead of using needles.

Personally, I wouldn't mind someone rubbing me with lavender oil for eight weeks, but we need a whole lot more studies before I can recommend it scientifically.

My friend, retired nurse Sharon Clearly-Leclair, gave me some essential oils to try post-flu. I applied some on my upper lip and ended up with burning nostrils. So if you want to give it a shot, make sure you avoid mucous membranes (eyes, nose, mouth, genitals). Sharon advises that if you have sensitive skin, mix your oils with virgin coconut oil before applying them.

SHOE INSOLES (ORTHOTICS)

Orthotics don't prevent back pain.[114] [115]

Nor have they been shown to treat back pain you already have.[116]

Unless you really love to spend money on shoe inserts, save your cash.

STOP SMOKING

There aren't any randomized control trials on smoking and back pain. It's not considered ethical to grab thousands of people and force them to smoke or not smoke so we can check if they develop back pain.

But we've done animal studies, cell studies, and computerized model studies showing that the ingredients in cigarettes can hurt your back[117] by drying out the intervertebral discs.

We've also done surveys on people with back pain to see if they're more likely to be smokers. Looks like it,[118] although it's hard to say for sure if smoking causing back pain, if back pain makes people want to smoke, or if there's some other factor thrown in.

Personally, I feel squeamish thinking about how rats and rabbits have been subjected to cigarette smoke until their intervertebral discs dry out,[119] [120] [121] [122] [123] [124] just to try and prove to humans that they should butt out. If you love animals, and you want to stop the pain, maybe that'll give you an extra incentive to trash the cigarettes for good.

DIET

This is about the only consistent thing that Western medicine has to say about diet and back pain:

Obesity correlates with back pain, at least for the top 20 percent of weight.[125] **So try to keep your body mass within normal range.**

However, that's not what most people are looking for. We all know that nobody recommends extreme obesity. The question is, can you change your food and drink in order to reduce back pain?

Answer: There's very little traditional research on this, at least not for otherwise healthy people in industrialized nations, because studies tend to concentrate on specific ailments like inflammatory bowel disease, or on certain geographic areas.

Let's talk about what we've got, which is **ultra low, level D evidence (animal and theoretical studies). No human studies at all. So if you read any further, just remember the following information has not been validated.**

1. Based on a mouse study: try to reduce advanced glycation end products (AGEs).

AGEs are created when fat or protein react with sugar inside the body. The big culprits are fried and fatty meat, processed food, and even high-fat dairy products and nuts. Basically, dry heat plus fat and protein are not recommended. So beware bacon and butter.

On the other hand, fruit and vegetables, fish, legumes, whole grains, and low-fat dairy products are A-okay.

Gee, where have I heard that before?

Yup, the American Diabetes Association, the American Heart Association, and the American Institute for Cancer Research all basically say the same thing: eat healthy food. Don't just grab fast food and instant crap.

Steam it, boil it, stew it, slow-cook it before you fry it.

Try not to barbecue as much (sigh), and if you do grill, add a citrus marinade, like lemon juice or orange juice, which will reduce the AGEs.

For babies, breast milk is lower in AGEs than formula.

If you want a paper with tables calculating how many AGEs per serving, check out this article by Uribarri et al.[126]

This is all based on a study that if you keep feeding mice AGEs, they'll develop spinal degeneration.[127] Mice aren't humans, so this is not considered hard proof in any way.

2. Based on theory alone (basically, no evidence): the alkaline diet.

This diet surged to prominence after Victoria Beckham Tweeted about it in 2013. It's supposed to raise the pH of your blood, which is normally somewhere between 7.35 and 7.45, mostly by eating fruits and vegetables, tofu, and legumes and drinking lots of water. You're supposed to avoid dairy, meat, eggs, processed foods, and most grains.

Reality check: your intake isn't really going to alkalinize your blood. Your body's job is to maintain a pH balance and it's darn good at it. Also, there's no clear evidence against milk and cheese, which help keep up your calcium and phosphate levels.

However, there may be some theoretical benefits to your health, mainly from eating fruits and vegetables.[128]

So I didn't find any good research on diet and back pain, but here are some suggestions from Dominick Hussey, an osteopath based in Ottawa, with comments from me:

a. Dominick: Stay hydrated.

Me: Always a good idea. Water is your friend. Almost any condition feels worse when you're dehydrated. Plus, chugging water makes you hit the bathroom regularly. Built-in exercise!

b. Dominick: Avoid caffeine. "Coffee makes me a lot of money."

Me: You always have to try things in moderation. So sure, you can cut caffeine out of your diet and see if that makes a difference. You can definitely save money that way. There are theories about why it might be a good idea to go caffeine-free, but I found exactly one article about it from 1997.[129]*)*

c. Dominick: If you have arthritis, avoid the nightshade family.

Me: Don't know there's any evidence about this. Again, no real downside to cutting out tomatoes, except you might miss the anti-oxidants. Try it and see.

In summary, traditional Western medicine doesn't pay much attention to diet, so rigorous dietary research is in its early days. Holistic medicine talks about diet without researching it.

If you want to change your diet, go for fruits and vegetables and avoid crappy, fatty foods. You don't want heart disease or diabetes anyway, and it may make you feel like you're taking control of your life in a way that taking pills doesn't.

GO OUTSIDE

Human beings are animals. We need to move out of our cubicles and into fresh air. This even has a name: green exercise. Exercising outdoors helps your mood, particularly for males. It increases self-esteem, especially in young people and people with mental disorders.[130]

Just five minutes outside can help.

Water is even more helpful, so if you can include a detour around a creek, river, or ocean view in your routine, it's worth it.

Going into the forest lowers your blood pressure, heart rate, and your levels of cortisol, a stress hormone,[131] and boosts your immune system.[132] "Forest bathing" or *Shinrin-yoku* is a tradition in Japan that is now becoming more popular in the West.

Can't go outside? Try a screen saver or a photo of nature. Just looking at pictures of nature, compared to pictures of industrial buildings, lowers your blood pressure in a stressful situation.[133]

Even though we don't have specific green exercise studies on back pain or randomized control studies, here's an interesting review article by Gladwell et al.[134]

TL;DR: When you exercise, you can probably get an extra boost from doing it outside, especially near water or in the forest.

RECAP

"Let me explain." Pause. "No, there is too much. Let me sum up." —Inigo Montoya, *The Princess Bride*

When we're in the middle of a Code Blue, one of the things we're supposed to do is to summarize what's already happened and what we plan to do. It helps keep the team on track.

So now that we've covered a lot of ground, let's recap.

You've got back pain.

SCAN: Make sure you move slowly, with your core, supporting yourself with your arms, and speak nicely to yourself.

Most low back pain is not dangerous, but get yourself checked out anyway, especially if you have any red flags.

Drugs: take them if you have to.

Start back on your regular routine as soon as you can.

Most people don't need imaging in the first month or two.

Acupuncture might reduce pain.

What you really need is exercise and education, **E2**. It helps for up to a year after an episode and may prevent the next one.

Walk, swim, do yoga.

Physiotherapists, chiropractors, Pilates, multidisciplinary teams, cognitive behavioural therapy and relaxation...they can help. They're not cure-alls. But what you really need to do is get moving and thinking.

You can try a bit of heat. Ice probably won't hurt.

If you like herbal remedies, there's some evidence for cayenne pepper derivatives, white willow bark, and devil's claw.

Things that don't have scientific evidence? Injections, back braces, insoles, TENS, lasers, ultrasound, lidocaine patches, essential oils.

Diets don't have any proof either, but you might as well eat fruits and vegetables instead of fried crap.

Buy the right kind of mattress.

Pay attention when you're lifting, and it wouldn't hurt to check how you sit, stand and walk, either.

If you want to get moving, and you want specific exercises that target problem areas, I'll outline an exercise program next before I get into specific diagnoses.

And then you need to get into your own headspace. Because this is not only a physical problem, but a mental and emotional thing, too. If nothing else, it's a mind game to go from perfectly healthy to even a minor pain problem, let alone a chronic one. So that's what we're going to finish off with.

GETTING IN THE MOOD TO MOVE

TYPE 1 & TYPE 2 FUN

I want to introduce the idea of different kinds of fun.

Type 1 fun is the kind of fun that instinctively feels good and almost everyone likes: hanging out at the beach, eating something delish, watching a movie.

Everyone likes Type 1 fun. But if that's all you get, day in and night out, it gets boring. It's passive.

Type 2 fun means achievement. Climbing a mountain. Obtaining a degree. Passionately raising a child. Writing a novel. Building a house.

The minute-to-minute pleasure quotient is not as high. You've got to put in the sweat equity. That doesn't always feel as good as, say, drinking tequila. But at the end of the day/year/decades, you look back and say, *It was all worth it.*

Turning your back around is more Type 2 fun.

For you, exercise may be Type 2 fun. No matter how much scientists talk about endorphins, you will not feel like getting out of bed every single morning. However, I want you to try it for at least four days.

FOUR DAYS

Four days are doable. They're not a lifetime of commitment. I'm not asking you to get engaged, get married, and have babies with an exercise program.

But try it for four days.

Why four days?

After four days, you start to make something a habit.

So give me four days. That's all I ask.

CLEAN SLATE

You're reinventing your life right now.

First, clean your slate.

It's easiest to start a new habit if you pair it with a new activity, like moving to a new place. That seems pretty drastic (and counter-productive, if your back hurts), but maybe there's something else you can do to make it new.

For example, start on a new day of the week. "It's Moving Monday. Here I go." Get a friend to join you.

☆ Print out some worksheets at http://melissayuaninnes.com/membership-join/ and put them in a binder.

This is the new you.

TREATS

Give yourself a treat every time you complete a set of exercises.

I mean every time.

Dr. Melissa's watching you.

Just kidding. But really, can you give yourself a sticker? If you're too cheap for real stickers (that would be me), could you draw a happy face on you calendar? Listen to a mind-bending song? Read a book? Poke around aimlessly on the Internet?

If you reward yourself for your achievement, you will want to do it more. That's positive reinforcement.

So if every time you stretch and strengthen, you get a treat, you'll start to think of exercise as fun.

Go for it.

Here are some treats that don't cost anything but can make you smile.

1. Nature
2. Laughing
3. Stroking a cat
4. Doodling
5. Sex

You get the idea.

Make yourself a treat sheet. Or write your treats right on your work sheet. That's how you'll stay the course, long term, until the exercise becomes its own reward.

E2 IN EARNEST: EXERCISE

10 REASONS TO TRY E2

I have to admit, when I pick up other back books and land on their pages of constipated-looking people exercising, my eyes glaze right over.

So here are ten ways my activity section is different.

1. You don't have to be perfect. You don't need flawless form or colour-coordinated clothes. You don't want to hurt yourself, but you can start moving intelligently.

2. You can orchestrate your own workout. If you already have an established program, ramp yourself back up to it as soon as your pain allows. I encourage you to incorporate cardio, core, strength training, and flexibility, but no one program has the magic key. Your back, as well as the rest of your body, wants you to move, and your brain wants you to be happy. If choosing your own activities makes you smile, have at it.

3. If you don't have a fitness routine, or this bout with back pain has inspired you to expand your range of movement, give mine a try. **I kept my plan simple.** Most people can do these exercises. But of course you have to use common sense, listen to your body, and consult with helpful professionals about what's wise to attempt at this moment in time.

4. You don't need any extra equipment or special training.

5. Begin in bed with exercises I call **Simple 7**. Uh huh. You don't even have to get off your mattress to start feeling virtuous and triumphant. ☆ **Download the worksheets** for all sets on my website.

6. Another big obstacle is that you're busy. So the next round of exercises is called the **Sneaky 7** because you're going to **add them throughout your day**. You don't have to carve an extra hour out of your schedule. You've got the same 24 hours as before, peppered with some extra moves.

7. Just before bed, if you've got enough juice, or this is the only time of day you've got to yourself, go for the **Sleepy 7** exercises.

8. Customize as needed. You're in charge. Every day, you decide what you want to do, and how much.

9. ☆ If you need more instruction, I've posted **videos on my website, http://melissayuaninnes.com/membership-join/**. Instead of watching some sixteen-year-old Olympian performing exercises with perfect form, you can admire Becky, who's doing the Simple 7 exercises in bed while her one-year-old son crawls on her. We're talking real life, not Photoshop. Real people with real lives doing realistic activities with real wardrobe malfunctions.

10. For cardio, you're the boss. Walk, swim, hip hop—as long as you're moving, and it's not hurting, you choose.

Q. How long is this going to take?
A. As long as it takes.

If you only have five minutes, give me five minutes.
If the next day, you have an hour, give me an hour.
I've seen other books that promise that you practically only need an extra two seconds per day, but then you're flipping past 2000 pages of exercises, thinking, how is this physically possible?
Answer: it's not. The amount of time you take per set depends on how much pain you're in, because more pain or more attentiveness means moving more slowly. Which is fine. And is different every

day. So the amount of time invested really depends on you and your body.

There are only two rules.

1. If something hurts, **hold on**. Remember, your body is talking to you, and if it hurts, that's your body's clever way of saying, "Don't do that!"

2. When the pain eases, especially if you can modify the activity in a way that works for you, **keep going**.

If you think you can go a little further, then do so. Your goal is to slowly advance, not stagnate. And if you stick with the plan, eventually, you'll get tired of hanging out at ground zero.

If you've had low back pain for more than six weeks, it's possible that your nerves have gotten into the habit of firing off even when you're not doing anything dangerous. The safest thing to do is to consult a professional about how to safely advance your exercise plan.

Every day your mind and body are evolving, and only you can tailor your activities to what you need. Part of your education is to listen to yourself and your body.

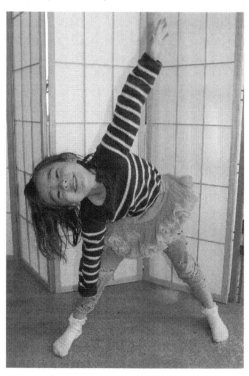

SIMPLE 7: MOVE IN BED

INTRODUCING SIMPLE 7 WITH PEAK POSE

It's morning. Yawn. You don't want to open your eyes, let alone get out of bed. Maybe you're already in pain and dreading the first twinge.

Good news: you can start moving right in bed. That's right, on your own mattress, maybe under your own blankets. Cool, no?

Just **SCAN** as you're doing it. Move slowly and steadily, supporting yourself with your **c**ore, with your **a**rms taking on more of the work, and treating your body **n**icely.

In that vein, if you need more firmness under your back, move to the floor or get a friend to slide a board under you.

PEAK POSE

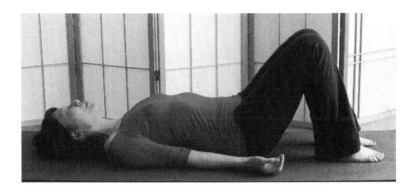

    While lying on your back, slowly bend your knees and tense your core muscles.

    Plant the soles of your feet on the mattress.

    See? That wasn't so bad. You can do this.

    This is peak pose. Your knees form a peak, like a mountain, or a triangle, or an electrocardiogram, or whatever metaphor most works for you.

1. HUG (KNEE TO CHEST)

**Goal: give yourself a hug. Or at least your leg.
Stretches your bum, lower back, and hips**

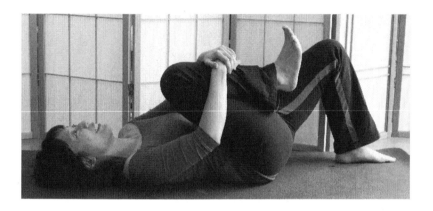

Start in peak pose.

SCAN. Tighten your core muscles, which means all the muscles around your midsection.

Press down into the mattress with your arms. Keep your left knee bent and your left foot pressing into the mattress while moving your right knee toward your chest and thinking of how awesome you are. If your mattress is too wobbly, you can move to the floor or another firmer surface.

To hug your right knee, you'll need your arms.

The left foot continues to press into the mattress. It's going to be the lying-down version of the arms, providing stability for you, while your real arms reach for your right leg.

Your core is your other secret weapon, also stabilizing you.

Hug your right knee. If you can't reach it, that's okay. You're aiming for it. One of these days, you'll touch it. It'll get closer and closer until you can give it a good ol' fashioned squeeze. In the meantime, you can loop a belt, strap, or towel around your leg and hug it that way.

Now you've got two choices:

1. <u>Dynamic</u>: hug each knee at least 4 times, and then finish off by holding each knee for at least 4 seconds, or

2. <u>Stability and flexibility</u>: aim to hug each knee for eight seconds or longer. If you're in pain, you may not want to keep alternating knees. You'd rather hold one position and work on flexibility. You can also try rotating your ankles or hips in circles while in this position, so you don't get bored.

Both choices are legit. They achieve slightly different goals, and you may want to vary your practice on different days. You do you.

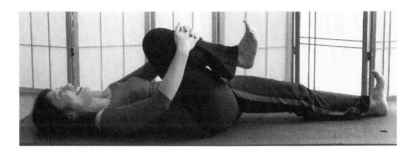

You may also decide that you're ready to leave your supporting leg straight out, on the bed or floor, as in this photo. If you've got it, go for it. If you don't have it yet, work toward it.

Alternative double hug: try bringing both legs to your chest at the same time. You will need core strength so you're not wobbling all over the place.

Whichever way you hug yourself, hooray! Huzzah! Champion!

2. GROUNDED TREE—>FOUR

Goal/stretch: fully open your hip and then your piriformis and gluteal muscles

GROUNDED TREE

Remember when you were in kindergarten and you got to pretend to be a tree? Either swaying back and forth in gym, or as scenery in the school play?

Yeah, I don't remember that, either.

Now you're going to be a tree on the ground. Still elegant, mind you.

Start off in peak pose. Your core is activated.

Now you're going to be a tree lying on the ground. Still elegant, mind you.

Start off in peak pose. Your core is activated.

Gradually straighten out your right leg with your left foot still planted in the mattress. Half in peak pose on the left, half with right leg straight. Right on.

Rotate your left knee out toward the floor.

Doesn't matter how far you go. What matters is that you're getting movement into your hips. Yee haw.

If you're a beginner, excellent. Hang out here for eight seconds.

Then do it on the other side (straight left leg, rotated right leg).

One leg will be easier than the other. That's normal. No judgment.

Physiotherapy calls this the classic FABERE stretch, which stands for hip Flexion, ABduction, External Rotation, and Extension. So this is a four-in-one stretch. Nifty, eh?

NUMBER FOUR

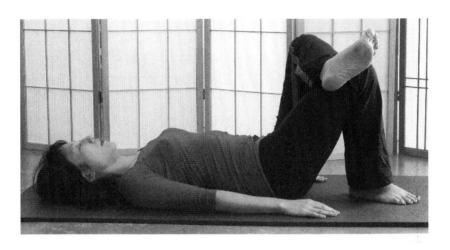

As your hip starts to open, you can move toward the number four.

That means you want to make the number four with your legs.

Say you're already in tree with your right leg straight and left leg bent.

Slowly, core-fully move your left ankle on top of your right knee. That might be enough for you.

If you still have some movement in your hips, start to bend your right leg, so that your right leg is lifting your bent left leg into the sky like an elevator.

Hoo yeah.

Eventually, you'll reach between your legs and hold on to your right thigh or knee. If you have trouble visualizing it, I posted the picture on <u>my website</u> ☆.

Whatever point you're at—number four on the ground, bottom foot planted, or holding on to your right thigh or leg, hold for eight seconds.

Change sides. Eight seconds.

Who rules the world?

YOU DO.

3. TWISTER

Goal: tip your knees toward the ground
Stretches the lower sides and back

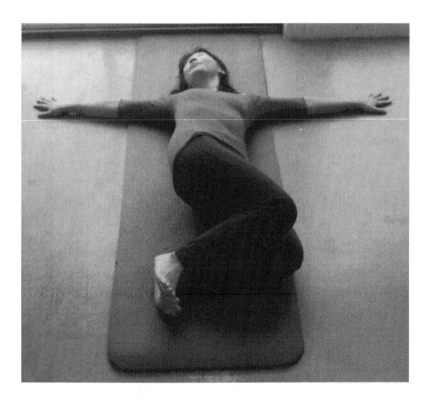

Back to peak pose, but this time, bring your legs and feet together so that they're touching. Yep, your thighs, knees, ankles and feet are kissing each other.

I want you to swish your hips a tiny bit to the right side, about an inch, then tip your knees to the left.

Your knees don't have to reach the ground, but tilt them as far toward the ground as you can without your back freaking out. You're aiming to hold this position for at least eight seconds. Again, that can be an end goal, but you're looking for mobility in your spine.

Bring your hips back to centre so you're doing peak pose with legs together. Lift your hips to plant them an inch to the left. Now try dropping them on the right side, gradually and carefully. Hold for eight seconds or more, according to your ability.

Again, one side may be easier than the other. Your body may tighten up and say, *Yep, this is the problem, right here.*

Good to know. It'll loosen up over the next few days or weeks. Linger a little longer on your tight side if you can.

4. ONE LEG TO RULE THE WORLD

**Goal: one leg up in the air. Bottom foot on ground/leg
stretched out.
Stretches the hamstrings (back of leg)**

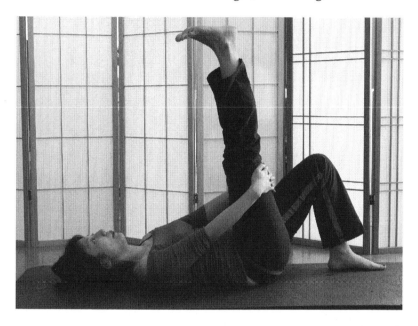

You're in peak pose again. Gotta love that. Ahh.

Now you're going to stretch your right leg straight in the air. Don't point your toes; keep your feet flat. (As yoga teacher Faith Hunter put it, "You want Ken feet, not Barbie feet, for this exercise.") Your core is engaged. You can also use a towel, belt, etc. to loop around the ball of your right foot. That'll keep the foot in the right place and help you reach your leg in the air if it's not happening for you yet.

If you're a bit stiff, as most of us are in the mornings, keep your left leg bent and its foot planted on the ground. It's the right leg that's workin' here first.

If you're feeling limber, don't use the towel or belt. Use your hands to hold on to your own miraculous right leg. Another option is to straighten your left leg on to the ground, pressing the back of the thigh and calf into the earth, while your right leg continues to salute the world, high in the air like a flag pole. Or like royalty, which is why it's called "one leg to rule the world."

Try to hold this position for eight seconds or more. If you like movement, you can slowly rotate your flagpole leg in circles, four times in each direction.

Gently lower your right leg to the ground and bend both legs so that you're in peak pose, using your core muscles.

Switch sides.

5. DRUMSTICK

Goal/stretches: the quadriceps (the front of the thigh)

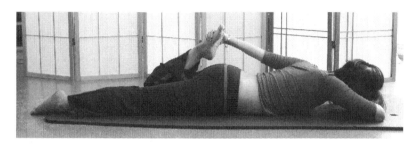

Roll on your side or on your stomach, whichever is easier for you.

Fire up your core muscles.

Grab your left foot, ankle, or pajama bottom. If you can't reach, loop a strap or belt around your ankle.

You should feel the stretch in the front of your left thigh.

Keep your legs relatively close together while doing this, i.e. don't let them skew off to the side too much.

Count to eight.

Let your left leg go.

Switch to your right side for eight counts.

6. YES, YOUR MAJESTY

**Goal: kneel with one foot planted in front and the other knee planted behind
Benefits: stretches the hip flexor muscles and front of thighs. Aims to reduce sciatica**

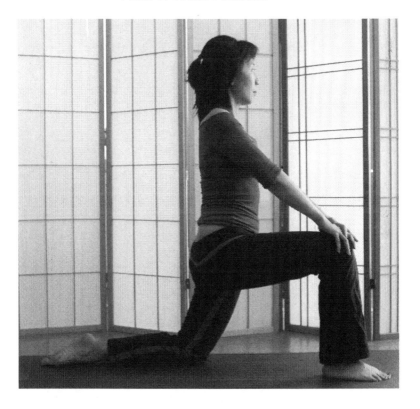

Core muscles ready.

Kneel with your right knee in front and your left knee behind you.

If you don't feel a stretch in the front of your inner thigh, either move your left knee back or lean your body forward a bit until you do.

But try and keep a 90 degree angle between your right thigh and your shin. It protects the knee.

Can you stay here for 30 seconds?

If you're bored, you can raise your arms in the air, which stretches out your abdominal muscles. Make sure that both hip bones continue to point forward. That is, if you had a headlight on each hip bone, they'd be shining straight ahead, on the same wall, instead of skewed off to one side.

Come down on your hands and knees before you switch legs. That's the safest way to do it.

And then kneel again, left knee in front.

For fun, pretend that you're being knighted. "Yes, Your Majesty. I shall serve to the utmost of my ability."

7. I AM NOT WORTHY

Goal: making your body into a 90 degree angle, bent at the waist and holding onto the wall.

Stretches the whole back, your arms, and shoulders. Hamstrings get a workout too.

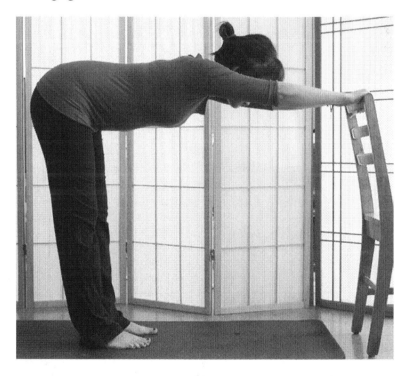

Okay, you have to get out of bed for this one. But you had to eventually, right?

You want to stand on a stable surface, so the safest thing is to use that core and arms and climb out of bed, congratulating yourself on being only one exercise away from *done*.

Stand a few feet away from the wall (basically, half your body height, including your arms).

Walk your way down the wall with your hands, core activated.

You're trying to get down so that your upper body is parallel with the floor and your lower body is parallel with the wall.

Hang out here for at least eight seconds, longer if you can.

In case you're wondering, I named this exercise after *Wayne's World* on *Saturday Night Live*. Mike Myers (before *Shrek* and *Austin Powers*) used to bow and cry, "I am not worthy!"

You're better than worthy. You're done the Simple 7!

For more exercises like this series, check out Dr. Gerard J. Girasole and Cara Hartman's excellent book, *The 7-Minute Back Pain Solution*.

SNEAKY 7: MOVE ALL DAY

1. STAND UP AND MOVE

"The chair you're in is a machine for producing human fat."
—Andrew Coyne

You already know it's no good to sit all the time. That means getting up. The good news is, if you're a year or two old, you already know how to do it. It's pretty easy to check "standing" off your list.

Next, *moving around* during your work day would be awesome.

"Oh, I can't."

Why? Because you'd look weird?

Well, just like in high school, you've got to choose between looking weird and risking premature death. I've always chosen looking weird, myself.

I think the dangers of inactivity are getting pretty well-known. Blocks your arteries, gives you diabetes and breast and colon cancer, and just plain cuts years off your life.[135]

So standing like a statue won't solve all your problems.

I remember when I was in med school, one of my classmates impressed everyone at a cancer surgery because he assisted for sixteen hours without needing a break. He said scornfully, "Doctors who *operate* sitting down, *pee* sitting down." I just looked at him and said, "Great. Both of those work for me."

Unless you need to get into a standing surgical specialty like that classmate of mine, non-stop standing isn't the best solution, either. Standing and sitting both put pressure on the discs in your back.[136]

You've got to move around when you stand up. If you drink lots of water, that'll force you to rise and rush to the bathroom regularly.

You're welcome.

Turn the page for six more ideas on how to move throughout your day.

2. LEG UP/TREE

Goal: stretch your hamstrings +/- hip rotators while standing. Also works on your balance.

Level 1

Shift your standing posture.
While activating your core, lift one leg up on a footstool.
Alternate legs.
You might have to get creative when you're doing this. You can use a stool while you're brushing your teeth or combing your hair.
I don't have a proper standing desk. I write on my dresser. So I pull out the bottom drawer and take turns which leg rests on it.
One neurosurgeon, Dr. Gerald Girasole, says he always sets one foot on the patient's bed rails while he's writing the patient's chart.

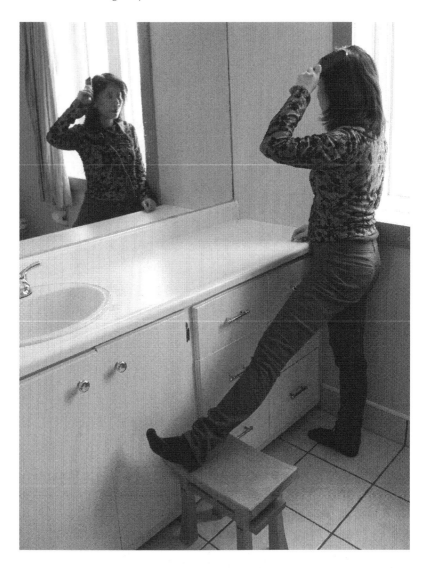

Level 2

Start to balance. Instead of the higher foot resting on an object, you're going to set just the toe on the floor. And then, as you grow more confident/cocky, you're going to start inching that foot higher so that you're balancing on one foot and the other foot is pressed against your ankle.

And then your knee.

And then your thigh.

Now, this is awkward to try with shoes on. You're giving yourself dirty pants. And you might feel odd. But I also find it liberating. Other people are just standing in line at the grocery store; you're balancing!

You may recognize this as Tree pose from yoga. You did Grounded Tree lying down on the floor. Now you're vertical. Fist bump!

You can hold on to something to support yourself while you're balancing. Eventually, you want to be able to let go of the object.

Because you're just that awesome.

3. TOUCH THE DOORWAY

Goal: stretches the side body. Lengthens and flexes the spine.

What if, every time you went through a certain doorway (say, your bedroom), you stopped to stretch left and right? Tighten your core and pelvic muscles. Use your arms to stretch out the sides, unless you have shoulder issues, in which case you can leave one or both arms by your sides.

If you lean toward the right, put a little more weight in your left leg, and vice versa. The doorway is a reminder to keep your shoulders in line with the wall instead of torquing them.

A doorway sway could take you a few seconds. No big deal, except you're getting a stretch in every time you go by.

You don't have to do it every time and get OCD (obsessive-compulsive disorder-ed) about it. But it's a reminder to get exercise in the interstitial spaces of your day.

If you don't want anyone to see you at work, try swinging toward each side before unlocking the bathroom stall.

Bonus: hold the stretch for at least eight seconds on each side.

It might feel weird at first, if only because you don't usually move side to side. But you're opening up your side body, which is pretty rad.

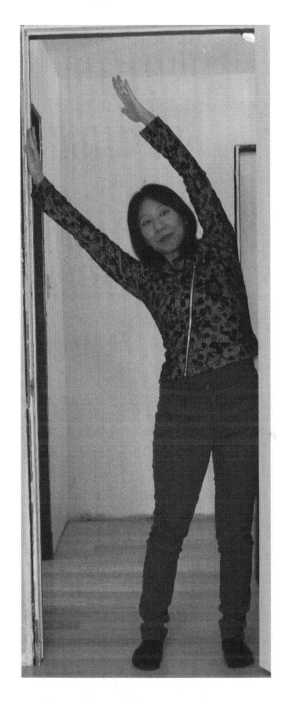

4. DYNAMIC CHAIR

Okay. You're going to spend part of your day sitting. So what can you do to get creative in your chair?

1. Foot stool

Keep a foot stool/recycling box/garbage can under your desk and alternate lifting one foot up on it at a time, stretching the foot stool leg out. It's like keeping one leg up when you stand, only while in a sitting position.

You get a hamstring stretch on one side and then the other. Make sure you spend roughly equal time on both sides.

If you've got a strong core, you can try lifting one or both legs up and straight underneath the desk. That'll activate your core and stretch your hamstrings. Basically, you're doing foot stool using an imaginary foot stool.

To make it easier, keep both your bum and your posterior thigh muscles resting on the chair. As you get better, you can inch your way to the front part of your chair. But not too far forward, 'cause you don't want to tip off the front of your chair and face plant on your keyboard. Not the way to win a promotion.

2. Seated '4'

Cross your ankle over your knee.

Bend your left leg and place your left ankle above your right knee. You can keep typing while you're doing this. Keep your right foot flat on the floor.

If you don't feel it, lean forward, back straight and core active. You should sense an opening in your piriformis, the muscle in the bum of your left bottom (side that's crossed). Hold it for eight counts.

Now straighten the left leg, bend your right knee and try your right ankle just above your left knee. You feeling it? Good. Give me eight counts here, too.

Feel smug about how much work you're doing, mentally and physically.

3. Half-lotus

I suggest you take your shoes off, because they'll get in your way. You may or may not be able to get away with this at work.

Cross your left leg and place the foot higher up on your thigh than in seated '4', almost in the groin area. You're stretching your hips, knees, and ankles. If it feels bad, back off to an earlier version. The idea is to have fun here, not injure yourself at your desk.

Meanwhile, keep your right foot planted on the floor like a regular person. Nothin' to see here, officer. I'm just sitting...in half-lotus pose!

Switch sides.

Try and work your way up to eight counts on each side. You can sprinkle half-lotuses throughout your day.

4. Cross your legs

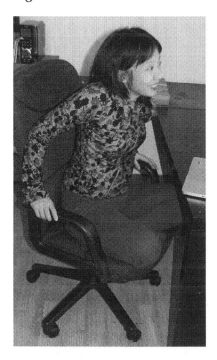

C'mon. Criss-cross applesauce one ankle over the other, and see if you can still sit up straight in your chair. It's like you're in grade school again!

If that feels too weird at work, give it a try at home. And make sure to alternate which leg goes in front. Only do this as much as your back tolerates. It opens up your hip rotators and your hip capsules as well as your piriformis.

The next few exercises start to require a bit more equipment, so they're optional.

5. Swivel it

You have a swivel chair? Ooh, aren't you fancy. Fancy in the oblique muscles, that is (the ones that help you turn your torso left and right).

Lift your feet off the floor. Hold on to your desk. Now start twisting your body from side to side. Try to do it eight times on each side, if you can.

This is the most amusing one, but also the most difficult to keep under wraps. Also, I just tried it and hit my thumb with one of the chair arms. But you're probably more coordinated than I am, right?

If you don't have a swivel chair, you can just turn your body left and right and back and forth like you've invented a new and bizarre dance. Or you could turn to the left and hold on to the chair arm/seat for up to eight counts. Relax back to the middle, and then hold on to the right side.

6. Ball chair

Could you swap out your chair for a big exercise ball?

This is a real dynamic chair. You have to use your core muscles to stay balanced, and it's just fun.

One of my friends had a ball chair in medical school, and I'd always call dibs on it so I could bounce up and down while we were talking about the best way to examine an ear. Highly recommended.

7. Bicycle

Some people buy little bicycle pedal contraptions to go under their desks that are so quiet, no one knows they're cycling all day.

I offered to buy one for my husband, but he said, "No, thanks." If you're more open-minded, you can give it a try. I might buy one for myself, because writing is sedentary, and my kids might find it cool.

5. PAT THE DOG

Stretches the back and the backs of the legs

If you're not in acute pain, and you're flexible enough, it feels good to lean over and touch your toes. Or pat the dog. Spreading your legs apart makes it easier to balance and makes it less stressful for the back.

I love patting my dog and getting in a stretch at the same time, but first you'll want to work your way up to that.

1. Face a wall.
Stand a step away from the wall.

Bend forward and place your hands on the wall, tensing your core muscles.

Walk your way down the wall until you make a 90 degree bend at the hip, while still touching the wall with your hands.

Hang out here.

That's right, it's "I'm Not Worthy" again! Because you love it so much! If you already did it, do it again, or cross it off your list. Yahoo!

2. Bum to wall.
Stand a step or half-step away from the wall—experiment with what feels good.

Keep your legs bent and your feet hips' width apart.

Press your bum against the wall. (Ooh! Feels good! You've got support.)

Slowly bend forward, away from the wall.

You can walk your hands down your legs if that's easier for you.

Let your head hang freely.

This should feel good, or at least reasonable, for your back. If it doesn't, you should back up, or get someone knowledgeable to help you ease into this.

3. No wall.

Legs hips' width apart but knees bent.

The wider the legs, the less your hamstrings and calves have to stretch. Do whatever feels good.

Bend forward at the waist with an active core.

You can touch your knees, your toes, or touch the ground. Bend your knees as much as you need to get here.

4. Pat your dog/cat/block/other prop

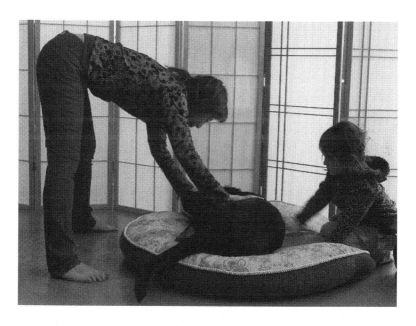

Keep a micro-bend in the knees. I don't want you blowing out your knees.

Bend until you're petting your animal/baby/phone/whatever.

Try to make this a little harder by bringing your feet slightly closer together.

Hang out here for up to eight counts.

5. Look, Ma, no props!
Ooh, look at you.

You can tighten your core, bend over, and touch your toes!

You could put nail polish on like this if you wanted! Guys, too. Why not? Part of keeping yourself limber. If that gets to be too much, don't be afraid to bend your knees a bit.

This one exercise that's going to make you and your pets ecstatic.

6. PLANK

The last two exercises, plank and triangle, are more difficult to do in public. I admit it. But the first one has the advantage that you've probably seen in it a meme. Do you remember when planking was a huge fad, like 2011?

I want to start incorporating a few core exercises here. But you've got to do them safely. So don't be shy about asking a physiotherapist, trainer, or someone else knowledgeable to check out your form. In medicine, the Hippocratic Oath begins like this: First, do no harm. I don't want to harm you. I want to heal you. But you've got to work with me. If it hurts, you may need a few pointers or some reassurance that you're doing it right.

Plank
Goal: you know how to do a push up. The idea is to **hold the push up position**, but first we'll start off with baby steps.
Benefits: core strength, back strength, arm strength, alignment of the neck and upper back, wrist flexibility

1. Wall plank/push-ups
Face the wall. Take a step back.
Plant your palms against the wall.
Lean forward so that your weight is on your hands.
Hold here for eight seconds.
Alternatively, do eight push-ups against the wall.

2. Desk planking
What's that desk doing there? Is there work on it? Quick before anyone sees you, back up a body length, set your palms on the edge, activate your core, and drop into a push up or two. Or eight. Or just hold here in plank, building up strength. Are you cool or what?

3. Half plank on the ground

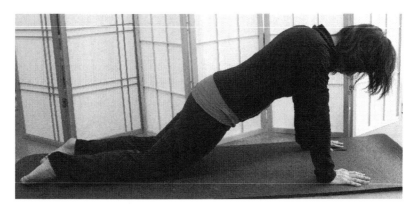

Get into push-up position, but on your knees. Palms on the floor, directly under your shoulders. Knees on the ground. Keep your back straight. You want a straight line from your head to your knees.

Your core is active. You can also tighten your pelvic floor muscles.

If you have any doubt, get someone to check your form, do it with a mirror, or place an actual plank of wood on your back. You can balance one end of the wood on the ground and the other on your spine. The idea is to hold yourself as straight as a real plank.

Hold here for at least eight seconds.

4. Plank

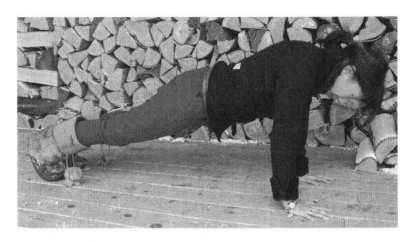

Knees off the ground. Arms straight and hands planted under your shoulders. Toes under. Body straight as a plank of wood (actual plank optional). Core active.

Work your way up to it.

7. TRIANGLE

Goal: stretch out your legs, hips, shoulders, chest, and your side body in a pose thought to **reduce sciatica**

Another genius move. If I haven't managed any stretching all day, I'll do a quickie version of Triangle.

Stand with your legs shoulder width apart. Your left foot pivots outward 90 degrees and your right foot pivots inward up to 30 degrees.

Bring your hands out to shoulder height. Both feet stay planted in the ground.

Lean over to your left side like you're stretching along a kitchen counter. Then drop your left hand down toward your left leg. Your right arm reaches up to the air. Your core is active.

Your shoulders are lined up in a single plane, so that if you were doing Triangle against a wall, both your shoulder blades would touch the wall. This is more important than trying to get your left hand closer to your right ankle.

To make it more comfortable, try bringing your feet closer together, or move your left hand higher up your left leg.

Take some breaths here, at least three, before you inhale yourself back up to standing.

You can let your arms rest by your side. Then raise them up again to try the same thing on the other side.

☆ If that explanation makes no sense, I've got a few more pictures on my website on how to get into the pose. Or look up "Triangle pose yoga" online.

I hated doing this pose when I started yoga. I always felt so stiff. But it worked for me, and now it's my daytime go-to pose. You don't need a wall. You don't need to touch the ground. You can just do your own thing. No one's around? Drop into a quick Triangle.

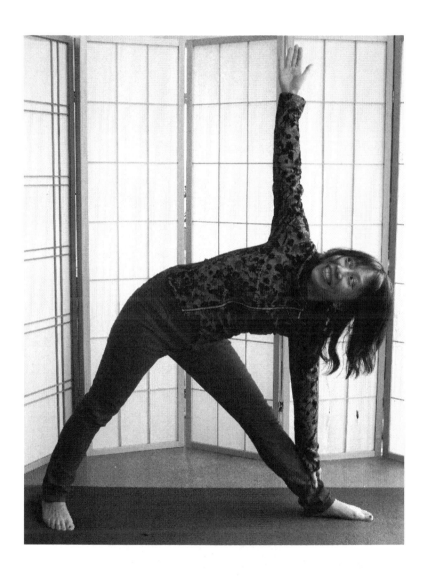

SLEEPY 7: MOVE AT NIGHT

1. CAT-COW

Please note these exercises are sequenced partly so they start off easily and partly so that they flow one into another. However, once you master them, you may want to rearrange them so that they end in a way that's more conducive to sleep.

Cat-Cow benefits: stretches and strengthens the spine and neck. Stretches the back, abdomen, and hips. Improves balance and coordination.

You worked hard all day. Now you get to be an animal. Two animals!

Get on all fours, palms under your shoulders with your arms straight but not ramrod-straight and your knees under your hips. Your core is engaged. Your back is straight enough to balance a wooden plank on it. That's **table pose**. And now, animal time.

COW

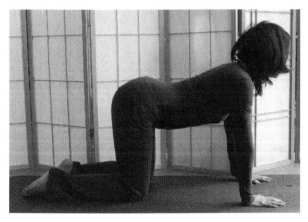

Inhale and arch your back. Curve your head upwards, so your gaze is climbing up the wall.

Meanwhile, your tailbones is also curving upward, so your most excellent rear end is shining upward.

Your stomach curves toward the ground.

Hold here for at least one breath.

CAT

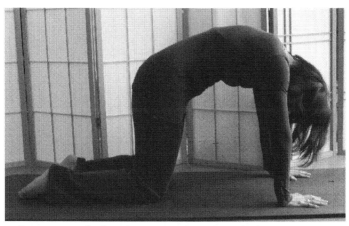

When you exhale, drop your head back down.

Curve your bum down.

Your core and pelvic floor are still active.

Your mid-back rises like a scared Hallowe'en cat, or like a sunrise, if you prefer more positive imagery. Think how slim and hollow you look from the side.

Keep changing on the inhale and exhale. I would say hip, hip, hooray if you could do four cats and four cows. I would start a conga line if you could do eight of each.

Level up: balancing

If you want to level up, come back to table pose.

Try extending your left leg in the air and balancing on the remaining three points. It feels weird at first, but if you use your core, you should be able to hold it for two, four, six, eight seconds (eventually).

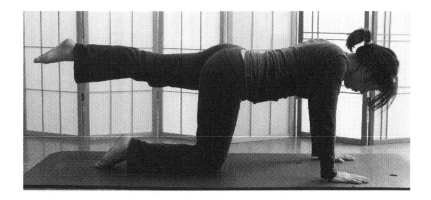

After this, switch sides so your right leg is in the air.

Level up once more: balancing on two points

If want an extra challenge, try extending your left leg in the air behind you and your right arm in front of you. This takes more core strength. You may wobble as your core builds up. That's okay.

The hand position is up to you. Personally, I usually hold my hand sideways and imagine that I'm shaking someone's hand, that someone is reaching out for me. Psychologically, for some reason, that makes it easier for me to balance. But you may prefer to turn your palm up, thinking that your palm is raised toward the sky, or turn your palm down, and imagine that the earth is sustaining you. All of them are valid options that may change from day to day.

Try doing four on each side, or simply hold each side for up to eight seconds.

2. CHILD'S POSE

Benefits: stretches the hips and ankles. Releases the shoulders, chest, arms, and back.

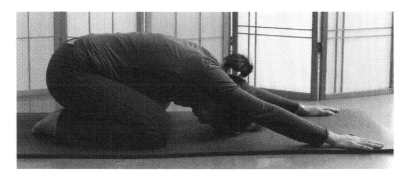

You want to rest, right? Me, too.

Well, one way to relax your back is to get into child's pose.

Kneel.

Sit on your heels. Or at least try and lower your buttocks toward your heels.

Then slowly, core-fully lower yourself down so that your head is touching the mat.

If you can't reach the mat, bring the floor up to you by placing a pillow or two on the floor.

Similarly, if your hips or ankles are the problem, put a pillow or block between your heels.

Place your arms either by your ears or by your sides. Your choice.

This pose should feel good. You should be able to relax like this. Like a kid taking a nap. Feel free to wiggle out your shoulders or otherwise adjust yourself.

Take a few breaths. Listen to some music. It's all good.

3. TV WATCHING

Benefits: lengthens and strengthens the spine. Tones your gluteal muscles. Stretches your abdomen, chest, and shoulders.

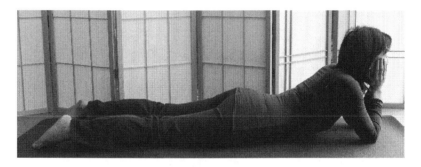

You want to incorporate a little TV into your night? How about doing it while lying on your stomach, with your chin propped on your hands and your legs long?

If you want to move, bend your legs at the knee and make circles with your lower legs, or tip them from side to side, always moving slowly and using your core.

If it's too much to lie down on your stomach, try propping yourself more up on your arms while you're doing it. The backbend will do you good. Pillows under your chest are an option if you need to work on your arm strength.

4. SUNTAN

Benefits: strengthens the muscles of your back, glutes, posterior legs, and eventually arms. Improves your balance and posture. Stretches your thighs, abdomen, +/- arms.

Nowadays, you're not supposed to get a tan. You're supposed to hang out in the shade and wear sunscreen until the stars are shining.

Since no one actually follows that one hundred percent of the time, this is a little somethin' you could do while soaking up some rays.

Lie on your stomach.

Straighten your legs behind you. Slowly, using your core, thinking how wonderful you are.

Now, keeping your core alive, lift your right leg into the air, keeping it long and strong. All your other limbs press into the floor, so you've got three points of contact and just one in the air.

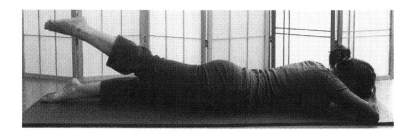

Gently lower it to the ground before you lift up your left leg. Do each leg four times each.

Level up

You're in the same position, lying on your stomach with your legs straight behind you, except you stretch your arms in front of you, so they're alongside your ears. Don't lift so high that your shoulders are cringing into your ears. You're relaxed. You're getting vitamin D.

Next, while engaging your core, lift your left leg in the air and your right arm at the same time.

Woo hoo! Now you're cooking with evil gas, as the Kids in the Hall used to say.

Lower your arm and leg. It's the other side's turn: right arm and left leg slowly, core-fully in the air. Keep your pelvic muscles active too.

Try four times on each side, for a total of eight times.

5. SIT TALL

Benefits: stretches and strengthens muscles of the legs. Strengthens back. May help prevent sciatica.

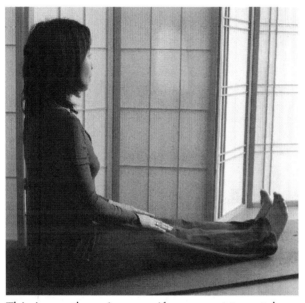

This is another nice one if you want to catch a movie or hang out while seated.

Try sitting on the floor with your feet stretched out in front of you. Straight-ish legs, back straight, toes toward the sky.

You're lengthening your hamstrings and calf muscles at the back of your legs. You're using your core to stay upright. You're practicing good posture, because it's hard to slump like this.

Most North Americans like to sit on chairs, but my ethnically half-Indian, half-Irish friend used to entertain with pillows on the floor so we could sit or lounge on the ground together. For some reason, it felt cozier than chairs. We could start a floor-sitting revolution.

6. BABY CORE & V

BABY CORE

Personally, I find core exercises super boring. So I don't do them. And then my core gets weaker, so the exercises get harder, and I don't do them...you see why this is Not Good?

Time to turn it around with baby moves.

Level A: <u>peak pose</u>. Lie on your back with your knees bent and your soles resting on the floor. Yeah! You already know this one.

Level B: contract your core muscles while you're in peak pose. That means tensing all the muscles around your waist. Front, sides, and back, like a superhero belt. Count to eight.

Keep breathing.

Tip: Once you get used to the feeling, you can activate your core throughout your day. You don't have to be lying down. So if you're waiting at a stop light, or in the midst of a boring meeting, work your core. First of all, no one will notice. And if they do, you just look svelte and taller.

Level C: Rock it into neutral

Say you're lying down in peak pose. Can you press your lower back into the ground? It means letting your shoulders curve forward a bit, because you're got your core activated and you want to push your lower back gently into the earth.

Now you're going to gently change directions and arch your back like you're a bikini model. Yep, even if you're a guy. Let dem headlights shine.

Slowly, of course. Still using your core.

Then let your back come into neutral. Somewhere between the two positions. That's where you should hang out in general. But you might have to rock back and forth a few times to get a feeling of that's neutral/normal/feels good for you. And it's a good idea to rock it anyway, and not get stuck in a weird position.

Again, you can take this to the streets. In fact, I encourage you to do it. Are you stuck in a boring lecture? Try arching and hunching a bit—not enough for other students to stare at you, but adjust yourself back to neutral.

V

Say your core is grounded and you're beyond baby moves. Go for V.

Benefits: not only strengthens the core, but stretches and strengthens the hip flexors that get so tight from sitting all day. Lengthens the spine and hamstrings. Strengthens the back. Improves your balance.

Level 1

Lean back from your sitting tall position. Plant your hands behind you. You've got your core going (don't leave home base without it). You're thinking of how incredible you are, exercising while everyone else is eating bon bons.

Come down on your forearms so that you can balance.

Lift your left leg in the air.

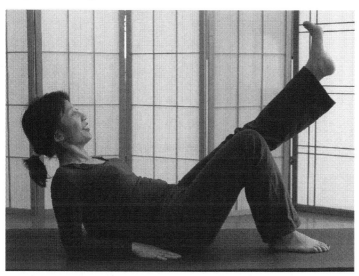

Put it down. Lift your right leg in the air.

Level 2

If that's super easy for you, try lifting both legs at the same time, still resting on your forearms.

Level 3

Take your arms forward, so your hands are gently resting on or behind your knees.

Balance on your sitting bones (your ischial tuberosities, if you want to look them up).

Lift your legs, but keep them bent at the knee.

Holding the backs of your legs makes this pose easier, because you get to use your arms as well as your core. SCAN all the way.

Level 4

Same pose as level 3, but straighten your legs, and your arms support themselves in the air, level with the floor.

Level 5

Straight legs and arms stretched above head.

No matter where you are, own it. Fabulous work.

7. BRIDGE

Benefits: stretch your hip flexors, tone your buttocks, work on your core strength, and get a backbend, all at the same time. #WorthIt #GeniusPose

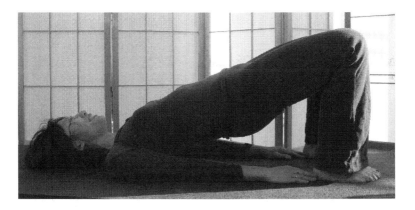

Look at you. You're almost all done! This is the last activity before bed.

First, peak pose with a difference: on your back, knees bent, feet planted on the floor, but you're going to move your heels a bit closer to your bum. Your feet should either be pointed straight forward or slightly inward.

Your arms are lying by your sides.

Breathe.

Inhale and lift your bum off the ground. Gently, using your core and activating your pelvic muscles, press your feet into the ground to stabilize yourself.

Gaze up at the ceiling instead of twisting your neck from side to side.

You shouldn't feel a lot of pressure in your neck. If you do, stop and ask someone to check your form and/or your neck the next time you try.

If your neck is okay, keep going. Make sure that your knees stay in line. You don't want them flying apart and making a diamond shape. Bring them slightly together, like you're squeezing a beach ball between them.

Raise your hips as high and as long as you feel comfortable.

Lower back down.

You can build up to three breaths and/or three repeats.

Now go forth and relax.

A WEEK

You gave me four days.
Now I want a week. That's only three more days.
You can do it. You're over halfway there.

BACK SLIDING

You didn't exercise yesterday?

Okay. Make sure you move today. And the next day.

Missed it again?

Try again.

Walking for a minute is better than no walking.

One exercise is better than no exercise.

When they study dieters, the problem isn't that dieters fall off the wagon. We all like to "cheat" once in a while because, let's face it, without the good stuff, life is boring.

But the problem isn't a few extra calories one day and then coming back on the diet. The problem is the dieter saying, "I blew it" and eating chocolate-peanut-corn chip-candy-whipped cream-beer-nacho-muffin-birthday cake supreme and falling into a permanent food coma.

So if you tumble off the exercise wagon, just get back on again. No recriminations, no big deal. Eventually, exercise will become part of your life.

A MONTH

A month. That feels good, to say, "I tried it for a month." That's a whole cycle of the moon.

Can you give E2 a month?

THE NEXT MILESTONE: 66 DAYS

Why 66 days? Because that's what at least one study says it takes to make a new habit.[137]

It may seem impossible, but once you make a new habit, it's ingrained.

It goes from "Just one more thing I have to do" to "This thing I do." It's part of your routine, like brushing your teeth. No big deal, except you feel better, and look better, and people stop you to say, "Hey, you look awesome. What's up?" which keeps you in the loop, especially if they join in too.

Hello, superstar.

I HAVE A DIAGNOSIS. WHAT DOES THIS MEAN?

"Knowledge is power. Information is liberating. Education is
the premise of progress, in every society, in every family."
—Kofi Annan

Okay. You know the basics of back pain and how to make it
better.

Let's say you've got a few more questions. You've got your MRI
report in hand and need a little translation.

I have a few words about some of the more common conditions.
I've put the explanations here because 85 percent of the time,
there's no specific diagnosis, and most diagnoses require the same
overall treatment (NSAIDs or other medications, exercise, and, for
a minority, procedures). But since knowledge is power, let's saddle
up.

DEGENERATING AND HERNIATED DISCS

The discs are the shock absorbers of the spine, the nice little cushions between the bones. Think of them like strong but flexible jam doughnuts sitting there.

A **degenerative or bulging disc** means that your doughnut is compressed. Someone is pressing on your doughnut, but the jam is still inside. It's usually not a big deal. Happens with age. This picture shows a very advanced case.

Osteoarthritis of Spine

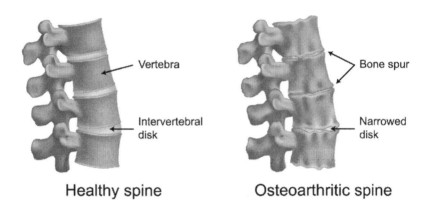

Healthy spine   Osteoarthritic spine

But what if those discs spring a leak, like jam squooshing out of a doughnut after you take a bite? (The 'jam' is the nucleus pulposus.)

Well, that's a **herniated disc, a.k.a. slipped/prolapsed/ruptured/ displaced disc**. Whatever you want to call it, a bit of squooshed jam. Too much jam can press on a nerve or simply irritate it by releasing chemical mediators.

But there's no need to panic. Lots of people run around with herniated discs and have no pain. (One in five people under the age of 60, actually. After age 60, it's more like one in three pain-free people.)[138]

How is this possible? Doesn't the all-seeing, all-knowing MRI tell you everything?

Well, not really. The MRI is a picture of your body. A sophisticated picture, but a picture nonetheless. That picture is not you.

Once, a doctor put up a physical X-ray film on a light box and asked the medial students how they wanted to treat the patient. After a student pontificated on the correct course of treatment, the doctor handed him a pair of scissors and said, "That's how you treat an X-ray. You want to treat a patient."

Sure, the jam may push on a nerve. Or it may just release hormones that irritate the nerve.[139] [140]

You can talk to a surgeon if you want. Just know that in the past, surgery[141] had the same outcome as conservative treatment.[142] In other words, long term, cutting people open had about the same success rate as taking anti-inflammatories and so forth. But it's your body, your money, and your recovery time.

And by the way, if the scan shows a **Schmorl's node**, fugghedaboutit. Those are totally benign (no big deal).

SCIATICA

This is a general term for pain associated with the sciatic nerve, the longest and fattest nerve in your body.

Because it's such a long nerve, symptoms vary depending on where and how the nerve is irritated. You may feel

- pain in your lower back or bum radiating down your thigh and possibly down to your foot, that gets worse with sitting
- numbness, weakness, or tingling
- difficulty moving the foot
- constant pain vs.
- shooting pain vs.
- burning pain

If you can't control your bladder or bowels, the weakness is getting worse, or you notice numbness spreading to your upper thighs, head for a real, live doctor, stat.

Sounds like a whole lot of fun, right? But everyone is different. Maybe it's something that only bugs you once in a while. Or maybe it's completely debilitating. Symptoms vary a lot. So does the cause.

Sometimes it's from a herniated disc, although studies show that it's less than 50 percent of the time. Other causes include spinal stenosis, spondylolisthesis, pregnancy, and piriformis syndrome.

Plus it doesn't help if you're overweight, not exercising, or wearing high heels.

TREATMENT

I'll say off the top that when I meet patients with sciatica/radicular symptoms, they seem to experience more pain that lasts longer, and it seems harder to treat than your average muscle pull.

Still, you start off with the same kinds of tools as with other kinds of back pain.

Drugs: you can try acetaminophen and non-steroidal anti-inflammatories, even if they're not as effective. Your doctor may need to bring out the bigger guns, like antidepressants, anticonvulsants, short-term muscle relaxants, or a very careful and limited use of narcotics.

Exercise: essential for prevention and will need to be integrated into your life as part of your therapy. You want to build a strong core and back muscles as well as flexibility. Gosh, I never heard that before.

Acupuncture: can reduce chronic pain

Physical therapy: In his book *The End of Pain*, Dr. Patrick A. Roth[143] states that McKenzie Physical Therapy was specifically designed for patients with herniated discs that cause pain on sitting. It works best if the nucleus pulposus (jam part) hasn't already broken through the annulus (fibres), and it may be too late if the nucleus pulposus is completely extruded. For that reason, he suggests an MRI before McKenzie physiotherapy to make sure that you'll benefit from it.

Steroids: I know I said there was no convincing evidence for steroids, either by injection or by mouth. But I also said that it's possible they could help some select patients. You could be one of them.

Cognitive behavioural therapy: can help anyone with back pain, but if symptoms drag on for months, therapy may be especially helpful.

Chiropractors: not proven to help long term, but if you have the means, you would probably want to try for even a short-term reduction in pain

Surgery: whether it's minimally invasive surgery to take out the bit of disc that's compressing a nerve or a full-blown spinal fusion, it's an invasive procedure, and you'll have to weigh the risks and benefits with your surgeon. Dr. Roth's book has some good discussion on this. Get a second opinion, ask questions like "How many of these procedures have you done? How much disc or bone do you remove? How do you protect the surrounding muscles?" Also, know that you'll need even more physical therapy after surgery than before.

PIRIFORMIS SYNDROME

The piriformis muscle is your friend. It helps you rotate your hip and leg out to the side when your knee is bent, like in the Tree exercise.

However, we think that in some cases (less than 6 percent of the time), the piriformis muscle can pinch the sciatic nerve, even though that's not often shown on MRI. Maybe your nerve is just giving off inflammatory mediators again, who knows. But if you look at Michael Teller's image of a dissected left buttock, you can see how piriformis lies right over the sciatic nerve (S).[144]

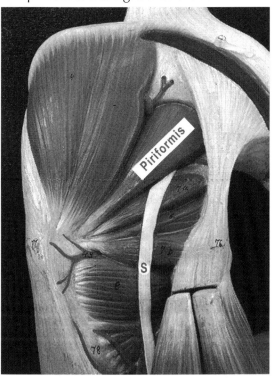

It's worth a try to stretch out the piriformis muscle and relieve pressure on the sciatic nerve with exercises like Hug, the aforementioned Tree, and Number 4, which are part of the Simple 7 Exercises.

You can also try rolling your piriformis on a soft ball. Tennis ball, lacrosse ball, a kid's squishy ball, whatever works. Or if you buy a foam roller, those work, too.

You don't want to roll the sciatic nerve and squash that. You want to rest your arm on the ground and your piriformis muscle on your ball/roller, gently applying pressure for about six seconds before you move on. A chiropractor named Donald Ozello made a YouTube video about it here: http://bit.ly/1WWmSwl.

SPINAL STENOSIS

So here's your spinal cord, protected by the nice little cocoon of bones around it. But what if the bones and ligaments start to push on the cord, like a fat kid stepping on a garden hose?

Well, if you're born with a big spinal canal (the hole for the spinal cord), you've got a lot more room to play with. You're okay. A lot of people run around with some spinal stenosis and never know it, because it's an aging thing, a common phenomenon after 50 or 60 years of life. It's also more common after trauma (car accidents, falls, sports injuries, all that fun stuff).

But if you're born with a small canal, the spinal cord can get pinched. The pinching **worsens when you're standing and walking**. You get pain, numbness, or a heavy feeling in your legs.

Shopping cart sign: your back feels better leaning forward, like when you're pushing a shopping cart, riding a bicycle, or walking uphill, because you're leaning forward and taking some of the pressure off the spine.

When you sit or lie down, the pain goes away.

That's a good thing in that, unlike a lot of back pain people, you instinctively know how to stop the pain. Sit down! Lie down! Awesome.

You can live for years with spinal stenosis and never notice a difference in your quality of life or in your MRI. In a small study of 32 people over 49 months, 70 percent of people saw no change.[145]

But you can end up slowly, unconsciously limiting your life that way, because if you stop moving, you stop living. So you'll want to stay as active as possible. Get on your bike and/or start swimming. In other words, engage in activities that don't require you to arch your back all the time.

Obviously, if you wake up paralyzed, or you can't control your bowels or bladder, see your doctor immediately. That's a surgical emergency.

At least one neurosurgeon, Patrick Roth, encourages patients to consider early surgery for spinal stenosis, before you end up sitting on your couch for the rest of your life.

Unfortunately, cutting at one spot on your spine might make the other vertebrae more unstable.[146][147]

So there are no easy answers, but we keep coming back to the same principles:

1. Stay active.

2. Try to manage your pain conservatively.

3. Consider surgery.

Unless your spinal cord is being squished, in which case, call 911 right now.

LOWER CROSSED SYNDROME

You have four muscle groups that aren't acting right. Two of them are too weak and two are too strong, probably from sitting all day.

The weaklings: abdominal and gluteal muscles

The tight ones: hip flexors and the back extensor muscles (our friends the *erector spinae, multifidus,* plus others I didn't mention: *quadratus lumborum* and *latissimus dorsi*). The hamstrings tighten up, too.

Some people call it distal or pelvic crossed syndrome.

I have to admit, most doctors don't tend to call it anything at all. It's something you hear more in the physiotherapy/chiropractic community. But it makes sense. Most of us are stuck sitting all day, and it throws the muscles out of whack.

So what do you do?

Same thing as you do for any other muscular back pain. Exercise, baby! Yahoo!

My exercise program will cover most people. But if you want to hone in on this specific syndrome:

1. Start off in <u>I Am Not Worthy</u>, which is a lunge pose.

Works the tight hip flexors

Let's say you've got your right foot in front and the left knee behind you. You've got your core firing. Lean forward a bit, although you still want your knee at no more than a 90 degree angle. You should still be able to see your toes. Do you feel pulling at the front of your left thigh? Those are your hip flexors. They're getting a workout. Right on.

If you're more flexible and don't have knee problems, bend your left knee so that your left foot is in the air.

If you feel like you can honestly go a little further, you can use a strap or a towel to loop around your foot.

If you're very flexible, reach behind you and grab your left foot in your hands.

But honestly, just I Am Not Worthy alone is a good pose. I've been doing yoga for two decades, but I've been sitting pretty much all my life, and I can feel the difference with that base pose. Lifting your arms in the air, as we often do in yoga, stretches out the abdominal muscles, but then I, at least, tend to concentrate on reaching and on balance. If you keep your hands by your sides and really listen to your body, you will feel this. You can also try moving your rear leg an inch back to stretch out its hip flexors.

2. Cat/Cow (Sleepy 7)
Works the tight back extensor muscles

If you can get on all fours, try curling like a cat and alternating between that and hanging out like a groovy cow.

But if you're stuck in a cubicle, or even an economy airplane seat, try the seated alternative.

Plant your feet on the ground. Keep your hands by your sides, or hold on to your desk—whichever feels most natural to you.

Exhale. Bend your head. Curve your back. Tense your core muscles. If someone's looking at you from the side, your body is making the letter C. And this isn't too weird. It's as if you're bending your head and body forward to examine a really interesting document.

Inhale. Arch your neck so you're looking up toward the ceiling. Stick your backbone out. Now your C is reversed. If anyone asks, you're contemplating an effective new sales strategy.

Exhale and bend forward.

Inhale and gaze ceiling-ward.

Repeat as many times as you can get away with. It may be easier to do a quick one-two several times an hour, or you may want to get away and really concentrate on cat-ting and cow-ing to the best of your ability.

3. **Active Abs**
Activate your core by tightening up your abdominal muscles. You can do this while you're typing, when you're washing dishes—any time, really.

Try to move your belly button toward your back. Don't suck in your gut and hold your breath. Just imagine like someone is pushing on your belly button and aiming it straight toward your spine.

You can also try tightening your pelvic floor muscles. But if that requires too many brain cells and coordination, just start off with your abs. Think of them getting stronger even as you're exercising your brain at work.

4. **Glutes**

a) Ultra-easy: while you're sitting, press your heel into the floor. You should feel your bum muscles contract. Alternate sides

b) Wall squats: stand with your back against a wall. You can start off with your arms by your sides. Or, if you're super excited, throw your hands in the air alongside your ears.

Keep your core alive.

Slowly bend at the knees until you feel a burn in your thighs. Your gluteal muscles are working too.

You can either work your way up and down like an elevator eight times, or you can hold the squat for eight seconds. Either way is useful.

☆ **Wall squat pics on my website.**

5. Bridge Pose (in sleepy 7)

Work your way up to this one. It'll be a challenge for beginners, and you often want your muscles to be warmed up instead of springing into it after sitting all day.

But it's one of those all-in-one exercises, stretching your hip flexors, extending your back, activating your core, and firing up your glutes. So if you're active and flexible and warm enough, it's a good one. Like when I first started yoga and a teacher said, "If you only have five minutes, do downward dog." In this case, if you only have five minutes, and you can handle it, try a little bridge.

SACROILIAC JOINT PAIN

Often seen during pregnancy. All your ligaments are loosening, but you can imagine that the ones in your pelvis especially relax, to make room for the *bébé*. 'Course, that means you end up with pain in your back and bum.

But they think up to 20 percent of low back pain originates in the SI joint, and obviously, not one in five back pain patients is pregnant. Sometimes, it's just one of those thangs.

Treatment: same plan as everyone else, except you can also try an injection into the joint to see if it helps with pain. In fact, this is how you might make the diagnosis, since the SI joint won't necessarily light up on imaging.

FAILED BACK SYNDROME

I have to admit, I don't see this diagnosis, except in studies.

But if it's yours, it's a heavy one to carry around. It means that you've tried everything and it didn't work. Yet.

The fact that you're reading this book means you haven't given up. I commend you. A lot of people would just say, *Okay, I got an 'F' on backs, that's it. I'm done.*

Maybe you've tried "everything"—multiple surgeries that didn't work, or only worked for a little while, or got infected and you ended up with even more pain.

Maybe your health care practitioners have told you they can't help you anymore.

You are not alone. In one study, 19 percent, or almost one in five lower back surgery patients had more than one surgery.[148]

Some people have lots of back pain, meaning both that it lasts a long time (over three months) and it keeps coming back, as in ten to fifty times per lifetime.[149]

Failed Back Syndrome brings up the question of yellow flags, mentioned in the Grade C section.

I'd also recommend trying the <u>Get Your Heart on Your Side exercises</u>. If they speak to you, you may want to try Dr. Sarno's *"Mindbody"* series. Or watch videos on how to how to release emotional pain, like this one: <u>http://bit.ly/1Slq80i</u>

I admit that this diagnosis is beyond my scope of practice. If you've had an army of people treating you, it's unlikely that an emergency doctor is going to swoop in and save the day. I can give you temporary pain relief, but unfortunately, it means you're going to have to return to square one and ask, Where is my pain coming from? What sets it off? Can I get down from 10/10 pain to 7/10?

In other words, that it's possible you won't get to a completely pain-free back. Sometimes more treatment makes things worse.[150] Sometimes the best you can do is chip away at your pain with exercise and education. You may also want to experiment with one-on-one tutoring, like at back pain boot camp/multidisciplinary rehabilitation, where they teach you to exercise and figure out how to work through and past your pain, as outlined in this NPR article (http://n.pr/1eTX82U).

SPONDYLOLYSIS

A stress fracture in your back. One of the little bones breaks off (at the *pars interarticularis*, to be exact). This sounds horrible, but actually, it happens even to kids, as in 5 percent of five- to seven-year-old children! And you don't see one in twenty kids rolling around on the ground. Not with pain, anyway.

You may notice pain in your back that gets worse arching backwards. Football players and gymnasts may be a little more prone to spondylolysis.

Treatment is the same as with regular back pain: find ways to move that don't hurt. Try anti-inflammatories. But if the pain lasts too long, you can talk a surgeon.

SPONDYLOLISTHESIS

Instead of your vertebrae being stacked on top of one another, kind of like a tower of blocks, one of the blocks slipped out of place.

This can happen with age, just with the bones changing shape and muscles weakening, often between the fifth lumbar and first sacral vertebrae (L5-S1).

Or it can happen because of spondylolysis (the previous diagnosis, the stress fracture), at the junction between the lumbar and the sacral vertebrae. This is the kind that's more common in young men and may not be noticeable. Again, the culprit is excessive back bending, so gymnasts and cricket players can end up here.

Symptoms: back and leg pain.

Treatment: children require their own treatment, so talk to your doctor about that. For adults: activity changes, NSAIDs. Selected people may require surgery.

SCOLIOSIS

You know what this is: an abnormal curve in the spine.

If a person bends over and to touch his or her toes and one side of ribs juts up higher than the other, that's often because of scoliosis.

Most of the time, it doesn't cause back pain. But a minority of patients need back bracing or even surgery, so you'll need to follow up with your doctor.

GETTING YOUR HEART ON YOUR SIDE

E3: ENERGY, THE MISSING INGREDIENT

"Success is almost totally dependent upon drive and persistence. The extra energy required to make another effort or try another approach is the secret of winning." —Denis Waitley

E2, exercise and education, will get you pretty far.

But there's one last piece. Energy.

That's why I'm calling the whole program **E3**: education, exercise, and energy.

You're more than a collection of neurons and skeletal muscle cells. You've got to *want* to turn your life around.

Reading, and even half-heartedly swaying your hips while reading, won't cure your back. You've got to get your heart on your side.

For some reason, Western culture is reluctant to talk about things that can't be measured or viewed under a microscope.

But in the end, that's who we are.

So this last section is about how to sift through the insides of your brain and your heart, which might help your back pain. I realize this may seem off-topic and weird to you, but it's only about 2000 words. What have you got to lose?

DO YOU THINK STRESS COULD BE HURTING ME?

People ask me this almost every shift. "Do you think stress makes my chest pain worse?" is the most common version.

They don't usually ask about back pain. But it's the same idea. Whatever is mechanically wrong, stress will magnify the pain for you.

And if people are telling me they have stress, it's because they already know, subconsciously, it's hurting them.

So yes. I think stress is hurting you.

Here's an exercise for you.

Name five stressful things about your life.

1. _____

2. _____

3. _____

4. _____

5. _____

MENTAL PAIN

"Mental pain is less dramatic than physical pain, but it is more common and also more hard to bear. The frequent attempt to conceal mental pain increases the burden: it is easier to say "My tooth is aching" than to say "My heart is broken.""
—C.S. Lewis, *The Problem of Pain*

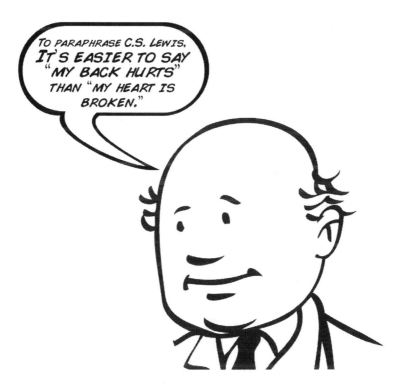

Is something going on here besides your back? Something else that's screwed up in your life?

Most of the time, the answer is yes, if only because life isn't perfect.

I first heard about this concept from Michael Crichton's book, *Travels*. When he was a medical student in the cardiac unit, talking to people after their heart attacks, they never said, "My cholesterol was sky-high, and atherosclerosis caused a 95 percent blockage in my LAD..." Maybe because that was before cholesterol became such a thing. Anyway, they'd always say things like, "My daughter ran away." Or "My husband had an affair."

In other words, they didn't view their disease as 100 percent anatomy. We could explain it in purely medical terms, and that would be technically correct, but it wouldn't tell the whole story.

If you want to get better, tell the whole story.

Think about what's hurting you in your whole life. Write it down, even if you have to buy one of those little diaries with a key or create a secret file on your computer.

Sometimes pain in the back is just pain in the back. A cigar is simply a cigar.

But sometimes, as C.S. Lewis pointed out, it's easier to blame your body than to try and make real changes like leaving an abusive partner.

Only you know what's going on in your life. And life changes, too. This back pain you're feeling now might be in your facet joints, but when it hits in ten years, it might get a little extra oomph because your son is moving to Antarctica.

If this speaks to you at all, give it a try.

Face your life.

Name one thing you hate about your current situation. Doesn't matter how big or small it is. Name it anyway.

1. _____

_____

FIVE THINGS I CAN CHANGE ABOUT MY LIFE

It's easy to run into naysayers.

It's easy to say, "My back hurts and there's nothing I can do about it."

It's hard to chart out what you can change in your life.

It's hardest of all to make the change.

But I want you to do it.

Little changes, like stretching your hamstrings every morning in bed.

Or big changes, like getting a divorce or kicking your job to the curb.

Five things I can change about my life.

1. _____

2. _____

3. _____

4. _____

5. _____

NO DISEASE, SHORT LIFE

"One disease, long life; no disease, short life."
—Chinese proverb

I first read this in a book called *The Tao of Pooh*, by Benjamin Hoff. And that was eye-opening, the idea that an illness could wake you up, shake you out of your complacency, and make you tend to your health and take your life more seriously.

A breast cancer survivor just told me, "My life now is better than it was before I got cancer." That's the opposite of what you usually hear.

Before you get sick, you take health for granted. It's always there and always will be. So it doesn't matter if you're working a dead-end job or if you're dating someone who makes you grind your teeth. Right?

Not so much, as your back is kindly reminding you.

Our culture loves to attack disease. Fight it. Beat it to submission. Kill it. And that works pretty well most of the time.

But what if your back pain could teach you something?

Chuck Palahniuk, author of *Fight Club*, wrote in his novel *Diary*, "It's so hard to forget pain, but it's even harder to remember sweetness. We have no scar to show for happiness. We learn so little from peace."

I know that every time life knocks me sideways, it makes me a more compassionate physician, friend, and human being. It's easy to dismiss people and say, "You didn't need to come to the emergency room. Just stay home and sip fluids." But if I catch the stomach flu and I'm bent over the toilet, retching, I always think, *This is why people come see me. Because it's so horrible!* (Which doesn't make me go to the ER. But I feel compassion for the parents who drag their children in at 3 a.m.)

If you were some sort of incurably healthy superhero, wouldn't you be kind of annoying?

> "Why hope for perfect health? Perfect health leads only to greater greed. Treat illness as medicine, not disease."
> From "Ten Guides Along the Path," quoted by Geri Larkin in her book, *First You Shave Your Head*.

I'm not the kind of person who says "Everything happens for a reason." Genetics, family, culture, and money all play a role in health and illness. And some things are just random. However, I do find it useful to consider what kind of meaning I can wrestle out of any situation.

Britain's former Chief Rabbi, Lord Jonathan Sacks, talks about the Bible's parable of Jacob wrestling with the angel. Jacob wrestles on, even when the angel throws his hip out of joint, saying, "I will not let you go until you bless me." Lord Sacks concludes, "And that is how I feel about suffering. When something bad happens, I will not let go of that bad thing until I have discovered the blessing that lies within it." You can read the rest of the panel interview here (the Dalai Lama says some nifty things too!): http://bit.ly/1nAHE81

Poet John Keats wrote in his letters, "Do you not see how necessary a world of pains and troubles is to school an intelligence and make it a soul?"

POSITIVE THOUGHTS

I don't believe that every single person can think his or her way out of back pain.

Nothing works one hundred percent of the time, and everyone is different.

On the other hand, your mind does affect your body. If you're about to give a speech, and your mouth goes dry, your hands shake, and your palms sweat, it's not because a sabre tooth tiger is chasing you. It's because the anticipation of the speech in your mind is having an effect on your body.

So if you can turn it around, and think positively and genuinely, that's another tool you can use to heal your back.

Not everyone can do this. If you don't buy into it, you'll probably just feel dumb. But if you can shift your thinking even ten percent, and bring down your pain five percent, I consider it worthwhile.

CHANGE THE WAY YOU TALK ABOUT YOUR BACK

One way you can change the way you think about your back is to use different descriptive words (adjectives).

If you notice, yoga and other sites focused on healing will use soothing, strengthening words.

If you keep talking about your back like it's a busted-up piece of crap, it's harder to notice when it's getting better.

So think of even one other word to describe your back.

Q. Hey, how's your back doing?
A. Actually, today it's [a little more] _____.

Fill in the blank.

strong
supple
flexible
broad
long
resilient
responsive
healthy
hale
hearty
vigorous
fit
recovering
mending
recuperating
improving
growing better

perking up
blooming
glowing
illuminated
appropriate
suitable
at ease
full of vitality
full of well-being

If you can, make up a whole new narrative for your back.

Rodney Yee, "the godfather of yoga," is excellent at this. He guides you into restorative poses. Normally, you wouldn't want to just lie around for 20 minutes or an hour, but he speaks so well, it's like poetry wafting its way into your ear while you relax. I'm specifically thinking of the restorative sequence here, episode 3: http://bit.ly/1Y01dn5

INVISIBLE SCRIPTS

Do you have assumptions that guide your life?

Of course you do. We all do.

Ramit Sethi wrote a blog post about it here: http://bit. ly/1wyMbG8. Indian parents may give their one air conditioner to their son so he can study in comfort, and then he in turn gets a good job to support them, making their sacrifice worthwhile.

Sethi pointed out some "invisible scripts" most Americans have, like "I work hard, so I deserve this nice apartment/a few drinks/vacation." Some of his readers posted their scripts, like "You have to have a car, even if public transportation is cheaper and faster."

I see invisible scripts all the time in medicine. In the olden days, it used to be "You're the doctor, so you know everything." Now it's more like, "I've got Google, and you don't know anything." You can imagine I'm a real fan of that one.

But I also see "I'm hurt and you have to serve me! Fill out all these forms so I can get paid for being disabled! Get me a cup of tea!" Or "This is all Edwin's fault, and I'm going to sue the company for every last penny."

Some invisible scripts are helpful. For example, I started dating my husband when we were eighteen, which makes me feel confident and loved, even in unknown situations. But lots of invisible scripts are damaging, or at least can work for or against you. Another ER doctor and I were talking about how, when an accident or illness strikes, a lot of people are shocked and can't believe it's happening to them. This may be a normal reaction, but as a physician who sees lives reversed on a daily basis, I'll testify that you can waste a lot of time and energy asking "Why me?"

In fact, at any time in life, the question is, "Why *not* me?"

We all get one life. And in that life, according to a Chinese proverb, you receive ten thousand joys and ten thousand sorrows.

It's easy to celebrate the joys. That's what Facebook is for, right?

But the sorrows—our society doesn't know how to cope with them, especially if the situation goes on for weeks or months or years. Friends fade away. Work falls apart. Money becomes an issue, which makes the sorrow worse.

I'm not offering you an easy solution. There is none. But if you've got an invisible script that's not working for you, now is the time to re-examine it and try to write a new one.

Since I'm a reader and a curious person, during my times of personal crises, I've sought out books. A lot of self-help books are cheesy and repetitive, so I make sure to comb through them and choose only the ones that speak to me.

And one good thing about a crisis is that it points out who your true friends are. It hurts to lose the superficial ones, but as one of my fellow students pointed out when we were talking about medical schools, "You only need one."

One true friend can save your life.

Your most important friend is yourself.

I have faith in you. You would not have picked up this book if you didn't want to write yourself a new story. You can do this.

Sir William Osler, a prominent Canadian physician, wrote, "Ask not what disease the person has, but rather what person the disease has."

You are not just a bundle of back pain from misfiring nerves and muscles and broken bones. You are a human being and the author of your own destiny.

CONCLUSION

PUTTING IT ALL TOGETHER

To turn your back around, you need E3.

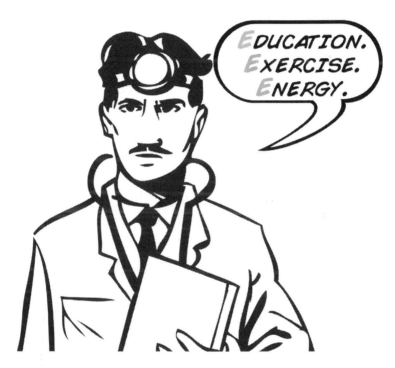

Education, you've got in your hands. But no book is a substitute for medical advice and lifelong learning. Explore http://melissayuaninnes.com/membership-join/ as well as other resources. Just remember to listen to your body and your B.S. detector, and you should be fine.

Exercise. I hope you start a program that works for you. Ideally, you'll stick with it for the rest of your life. But if it's something like quitting smoking and you have to keep circling around it and coming back to it, that's okay, too.

Energy, enthusiasm, willpower, spirit, fire, passion...whatever you want to call it, you need to put your heart into your health. As Helen Keller pointed out, "The best and most beautiful things in the world cannot be seen or even touched—they must be felt with the heart."

"Healing is a matter of time, but it is sometimes also a matter of opportunity." —Hippocrates

AUTHOR'S NOTE

"Healing may not be so much about getting better,
as about letting go of everything that isn't you—all of the
expectations, all of the beliefs—and becoming who you are."
—Rachel Naomi Remen

"You're going to write a book on back pain?" asked my friend
and internal medicine doctor Renée Givari.

"Sure! How hard could it be?" I said.

Pretty darn hard, actually.

Thank you to Lyn Worthen for editing.

Dr. John Beuerle, Dr. Joanne Bourcier, and yoga teacher Joseline
Beaulieu were kind enough to offer feedback on the manuscript,
but all errors are my own.

If you're having pain now, or you want to prevent it in the
future, I salute you. This is not an easy road.

"Healing takes courage, and we all have courage,
even if we have to dig a little to find it." —Tori Amos

ENDNOTES

1   Deyo RA, Tsui-Wu YJ. Descriptive epidemiology of low-back pain and its related medical care in the United States. Spine. 1987; 12:264.

2   Cassidy JD, Carroll LJ, Côté P. The Saskatchewan health and back pain survey. The prevalence of low back pain and related disability in Saskatchewan adults. Spine. 1998; 23:1860.

3   Coste J, Delecoeuillerie G, Cohen de Lara A, Le Parc JM, Paolaggi JB. Clinical course and prognostic factors in acute low back pain: an inception cohort study in primary care practice. BMJ. 1994;308(6928):577.

4   Deyo RA, Weinstein JN. Low back pain. N Engl J Med 2001;344: 363-70.

5   Hagen KB, Hilde G, Jamtvedt G, Winnem M. Bed rest for acute low-back pain and sciatica. Cochrane Database Syst Rev 2004; :CD001254.

6   Back Pain. David Della-Giustina MD interviewed by Mizuho Spangler DO. EM:RAP November 2013: 13(11).

7   Vroomen PC, de Krom MC, Knottnerus JA. Predicting the outcome of sciatica at short-term follow-up. Br J Gen Pract. 2002;52(475):119.

8   Bozzao A, Gallucci M, Masciocchi C et al. Lumbar disk herniation: MR imaging assessment of natural history in patients treated without surgery. Radiology. 1992;185(1):135.

9   Delauche-Cavallier MC, Budet C, Laredo JD et al. Lumbar disc herniation. Computed tomography scan changes after conservative treatment of nerve root compression. Spine. 1992;17(8):927.

10   Frymoyer JW. Back pain and sciatica. N Engl J Med. 1988;318(5):291.

11   Della-Giustina D. Back Pain. Interview by Mizuho

Spangler DO. EM:RAP November 2013: 13(11).

12   Ibid

13   https://breakingmuscle.com/strength-conditioning/at-the-core-of-it-creating-strength-and-tension-in-the-body

14   https://www.flickr.com/photos/michael_teller/4409149513/in/album-72157623429984269/

15   Harris RI, Macnab I. Structural changes in the lumbar intervertebral discs; their relationship to low back pain and sciatica. J Bone Joint Surg Br. 1954 May. 36-B(2):304-22.

16   McRae DL. Asymptomatic intervertebral disc protrusions. Acta radiol. 1956 Jul-Aug. 46(1-2):9-27.

17   Putti V. New conceptions in the pathogenesis of sciatic pain. Lancet. 1927. 2:53-60.

18   Lumbosacral Facet Syndrome Clinical Presentation. http://emedicine.medscape.com/article/94871-clinical

19   Stern J. Ending Back Pain: 5 Powerful Steps to Diagnose, Understand, and Treat Your Ailing Back. 1st edition. New York: Avery, 2014.

20   Deyo RA, Weinstein JN. Low back pain. N Engl J Med 2001;344: 363-70.

21   Ibid; cited in EMPH (2015) 2015 (1): 2-3. doi: 10.1093/emph/eou034

22   Casazza BA. Diagnosis and treatment of acute low back pain. Am Fam Physician. 2012 Feb 15;85(4):343-50.

23   Hagen, KB., Gro J, Gunvor H, Winnem MF. "The Updated Cochrane Review of Bed Rest for Low Back Pain and Sciatica." Spine 30, no. 5 (March 1, 2005): 542–46.

24   Malmivaara A, Hakkinen V, Aro T, et al. Treatment of acute low back pain: bed rest, exercises, or ordinary activity? N Engl J Med 1995;332:351. [PubMed]

25   Williams CM, Maher CG, Latimer J, et al. Efficacy of paracetamol for acute low-back pain: a double-blind, randomised controlled trial. Lancet. 2014;384(9954):1586–1596

26   Roelofs PDDM, Deyo RA, Koes BW, et al. Non-steroidal anti-inflammatory drugs for low back pain. Cochrane Database of Systematic Reviews 2008, Issue 1. Art. No.: CD000396. DOI: 10.1002/14651858.CD000396.pub3

27   Ibid

28   Muehlbacher M, Nickel MK, Kettler C, et al.

Topiramate in treatment of patients with chronic low back pain: a randomized, double-blind, placebo-controlled study. Clin J Pain. 2006;22(6):526–531

29   Yildirim K, Sisecioglu M, Karatay S, et al. The effectiveness of gabapentin in patients with chronic radiculopathy. Pain Clinic2003;15:213-8.

30   Staiger TO1, Gaster B, Sullivan MD, Deyo RA. Systematic review of antidepressants in the treatment of chronic low back pain. Spine. 2003 Nov 15;28(22):2540-5.

31   Salerno SM, Browning R, Jackson JL. The effect of antidepressant treatment on chronic back pain: a meta-analysis. Arch Intern Med. 2002; 162:19-24. PubMed

32   Skljarevski V1, Ossanna M, Liu-Seifert H, et al. A double-blind, randomized trial of duloxetine versus placebo in the management of chronic low back pain. Eur J Neurol. 2009 Sep;16(9):1041-8. doi: 10.1111/j.1468-1331.2009.02648.x. Epub 2009 May 12.

33   Goldberg, H et al. Oral steroids for acute radiculopathy due to a herniated
lumbar disk: a randomized clinical trial. JAMA. 2015 May 19;313(19):1915-23. PMID: 25988461

34   Hoppe JA, Kim H, Heard K. Association of Emergency Department Opioid Initiation With Recurrent Opioid Use. Ann Emerg Med. 2015 May;65(5):493-499. PMID: 25534654

35   Schnitzer TJ, Gray WL, Paster RZ, Kamin M. Efficacy of tramadol in treatment of chronic low back pain. J Rheumatol. 2000; 27:772-8. PubMed

36   Last AR, Hulbert K. Chronic low back pain: evaluation and management. Am Fam Physician. 2009 Jun 15;79(12):1067-74. Accessed February 1, 2016. http://www.aafp.org/afp/2009/0615/ p1067.html.

37   Casazza BA. Diagnosis and treatment of acute low back pain. Am Fam Physician. 2012 Feb 15;85(4):343-50.

38   Herndon CM, Zoberi KS, Gardner BJ.
Common questions about chronic low back pain. Am Fam Physician. 2015 May 15;91(10):708-14.
http://www.aafp.org/afp/2015/0515/p708.html#afp20150515p708-b28.

39   Chou R, Fu R, Carrino JA, Deyo RA. Imaging strategies

for low-back pain: systematic review and meta-analysis. Lancet. 2009;373(9662):463.

40   Jarvik JG, Gold LS, Comstock BA et al. Association of early imaging for back pain with clinical outcomes in older adults. JAMA. 2015 Mar;313(11):1143-53.

41   Shin JS, Ha IH, et al. Effects of motion style acupuncture treatment in acute low back pain patients with severe disability: a multicenter, randomized, controlled, comparative effectiveness trial. Pain. 2013 Jul;154(7):1030-7. Epub 2013 Mar 15.

42   Kalauokalani D, Cherkin DC, Sherman KJ et al. Lessons from a trial of acupuncture and massage for low back pain: patient expectations and treatment effects. Spine (Phila Pa 1976). 2001;26(13):1418

43   Vickers AJ, Cronin AM, Maschino AC, et al. Acupuncture Trialists' Collaboration Acupuncture for chronic pain: individual patient data meta-analysis. Arch Intern Med. 2012;172:1444–1453.

44   Chou R, Qaseem A, Snow V, et al. Clinical Efficacy Assessment Subcommittee of the American College of Physicians; American College of Physicians; American Pain Society Low Back Pain Guidelines Panel Diagnosis and treatment of low back pain: a joint clinical practice guideline from the American College of Physicians and the American Pain Society. Ann Intern Med. 2007;147:478–491.

45   Berman BM, Langevin HM, Witt CM, et al. Acupuncture for chronic low back pain. N Engl J Med. 2010;363:454–461.

46   Last AR, Hulbert K. Chronic low back pain: evaluation and management. Am Fam Physician. 2009 Jun 15;79(12):1067-74.

47   Barnes PM, Bloom B, Nahin RL, et al. Complementary and alternative medicine use among adults and children: United States, 2007. Natl Health Stat Report. 2008;10:1–23.

48   Steffens D, Maher CG, Pereira LS, et al. Prevention of Low Back Pain: A Systematic Review and Meta-analysis. JAMA Intern Med. 2016 Jan 11:1-10. doi: 10.1001/jamainternmed.2015.7431. [Epub ahead of print]

49   Rainville J, Hartigan C, Martinez E, et al. Exercise as a treatment for chronic low back pain. The Spine Journal. 2004 Jan 4(1):106-115

50   Carey TS, Freburger JK. Exercise and the Prevention of Low Back Pain: Ready for Implementation. JAMA Intern Med. 2016;176(2):208-209. doi:10.1001/jamainternmed.2015.7636.

51   O'Connor, SR, Tully MA, Ryan B, et al. Walking Exercise for Chronic Musculoskeletal Pain: Systematic Review and Meta-Analysis. Arch Phys Med Rehabil. 2015 Apr 96(4): 724–34.e3. doi:10.1016/j.apmr.2014.12.003.

52   Hendrick P, Te Wake AM, Tikkisetty AS, et al. The effectiveness of walking as an intervention for low back pain: a systematic review. European Spine Journal. 2010;19(10):1613-1620. doi:10.1007/s00586-010-1412-z.

53   Baena-Beato PÁ1, Artero EG, Arroyo-Morales M, et al. Aquatic therapy improves pain, disability, quality of life, body composition and fitness in sedentary adults with chronic low back pain. A controlled clinical trial. Clin Rehabil. 2014 Apr;28(4):350-60. doi: 10.1177/0269215513504943. Epub 2013 Oct 31.

54   Waller B1, Lambeck J, Daly D. Therapeutic aquatic exercise in the treatment of low back pain: a systematic review. Clin Rehabil. 2009 Jan;23(1):3-14. doi: 10.1177/0269215508097856.

55   Verrastro G. Yoga as Therapy: When Is It Helpful? The Journal of Family Practice. 2014, 63(9):E1-6

56   Cramer H, Lauche R, Haller H, & Dobos G. A systematic review and meta-analysis of yoga for low back pain. The Clinical Journal of Pain. 2013; 29(5), 450–460. http://doi.org/10.1097/AJP.0b013e31825e1492

57   Sherman KJ, Cherkin DC, Erro J, et al. Comparing yoga, exercise, and a self-care book for chronic low back pain: a randomized, controlled trial. Ann Intern Med. 2005;143:849-856

58   Posadzki P, Ernst E. Yoga for low back pain: a systematic review of randomized clinical trials. Clin Rheumatol. 2011;30:1257-1262.

59   Cramer H, Lauche R, Haller H, et al. A systematic review and meta-analysis of yoga for low back pain. Clin J Pain. 2013;29:450-460.

60   Chou R, Huffman LH; American Pain Society; American College of Physicians. Nonpharmacologic therapies for acute and chronic low back pain: a review of the evidence for an American Pain Society/American College of Physicians clinical practice

guideline. Ann Intern Med. 2007;147:492-504.

61   McCall MC, Ward A, Roberts NW, Heneghan C. Overview of Systematic Reviews: Yoga as a Therapeutic Intervention for Adults with Acute and Chronic Health Conditions. Evidence-based Complementary and Alternative Medicine : eCAM. 2013;2013:945895. doi:10.1155/2013/945895.

62   Yamato, TP, Maher CG, Saragiotto BT, et al. Pilates for Low Back Pain. In Cochrane Database of Systematic Reviews, edited by The Cochrane Collaboration. Chichester, UK: John Wiley & Sons, Ltd, 2015. http://doi.wiley. com/10.1002/14651858.CD010265.pub2.

63   Machado LA, de Souza MS, Ferreira PH, Ferreira ML. The McKenzie method for low back pain: a systematic review of the literature with a meta-analysis approach. Spine. 2006;31(9):E254–E262.

64   Machado LA, Maher CG, Herbert RD, Clare H, McAuley JH. The effectiveness of the McKenzie method in addition to first-line care for acute low back pain: a randomized controlled trial. BMC Med. 2010;8:10.

65   Ibid, Machado et al. 2010, BMJ.

66   Rubinstein SM, van Middelkoop M, Assendelft WJ, de Boer MR, van Tulder MW. Spinal manipulative therapy for chronic low-back pain. Cochrane Database Syst Rev. 2011;(2):CD008112.

67   Casazza BA. Diagnosis and treatment of acute low back pain. Am Fam Physician. 2012 Feb 15;85(4):343-50.

68   Walker BF, French SD, Grant W, Green S. A Cochrane review of combined chiropractic interventions for low-back pain. Spine (Phila Pa 1976). 2011 Feb 1;36(3):230-42. doi: 10.1097/BRS.0b013e318202ac73.

69   Cherkin DC, Deyo RA, Battié M, Street J, Barlow W. A comparison of physical therapy, chiropractic manipulation, and provision of an educational booklet for the treatment of patients with low back pain. N Engl J Med. 1998 Oct 8;339(15):1021-9.

70   Chen WL et al. Vertebral artery dissection and cerebellar infarction following chiropractic manipulation. Emergency Medicine Journal 23.1 (2006): e01-e01.

71   Norris JW, Beletsky V, Nadareishvili ZG, on behalf of the

Canadian Stroke Consortium. Sudden neck movement and cervical artery dissection. CMAJ 2000; 163(1):38-40. http://www.cmaj.ca/content/163/1/38.full.pdf

72   Karjalainen K, Malmivaara A, van Tulder M, et al. Multidisciplinary bio-psychosocial rehabilitation for subacute low back pain among working age adults. Cochrane Database Syst Rev. 2003;(2):CD002193.

73   Vollenbroek-Hutten MM, Hermens HJ, Wever D, et al. Differences in outcome of a multidisciplinary treatment between subgroups of chronic low back pain patients defined using two multiaxial assessment instruments: the multidimensional pain inventory and lumbar dynamometry. Clin Rehabil. 2004;18(5):566–579.

74   Stern J. Ending Back Pain: 5 Powerful Steps to Diagnose, Understand, and Treat Your Ailing Back. 1st edition. New York: Avery, 2014.

75   Schatzberg, AF & Nemeroff CB. The American Psychiatric Publishing Textbook of Psychopharmacology. American Psychiatric Pub. 2009.

76   Henschke N, Ostelo RW, van Tulder, et al. Behavioural treatment for chronic low-back pain. In Cochrane Database of Systematic Reviews. 2010 John Wiley & Sons, Ltd.

77   Casazza BA. Diagnosis and treatment of acute low back pain. Am Fam Physician. 2012 Feb 15;85(4):343-50.

78   French SD, Cameron M, Walker BF, et al. Superficial heat or cold for low back pain. Cochrane Database Syst Rev 2006

79   National Institute of Neurological Disorders and Stroke Low Back Pain Sheet. http://www.ninds.nih.gov/disorders/backpain/detail_backpain.htm

80   Roth, P. 2014. The End of Back Pain: Access Your Hidden Core to Heal Your Body (1st edition). New York: HarperOne, p. 177

81   Last AR, Hulbert K. Chronic low back pain: evaluation and management.
Am Fam Physician. 2009 Jun 15;79(12):1067-74. http://www.aafp.org/afp/2009/0615/p1067.html.

82   Oltean H, Robbins C, van Tulder MW, et al. 2014. Herbal medicine for low-back pain. In The Cochrane Collaboration (Ed.), Cochrane Database of Systematic Reviews. Chichester,

UK: John Wiley & Sons, Ltd. Retrieved from http://doi.wiley.com/10.1002/14651858.CD004504.pub4

83   Golish SR1, Hanna LS, Bowser RP, et al. Outcome of lumbar epidural steroid injection is predicted by assay of a complex of fibronectin and aggrecan from epidural lavage. Spine. 2011 Aug 15;36(18):1464-9. doi: 10.1097/BRS.0b013e3181f40e88.

84   Wong CSM & Wong SHS. A New Look at Trigger Point Injections. Anesthesiology Research and Practice, 2012, 492452. http://doi.org/10.1155/2012/492452

85   Staal JB, de Bie R, de Vet HC, et al. Injection therapy for subacute and chronic low-back pain. Cochrane Database Syst Rev. 2008;(3):CD001824.

86   Ibid

87   DePalma MJ, Slipman CW. Evidence-informed management of chronic low back pain with epidural steroid injections. Spine J. 2008;8(1):45–55.

88   Ibid

89   Ibid

Kapural L, Mekhail N, Bena J, et al. Value of the magnetic resonance imaging in patients with painful lumbar spinal stenosis (LSS) undergoing lumbar epidural steroid injections. Clin J Pain. 2007;23(7):571–575.

90   Dagenais S, Yelland MJ, Del Mar C, Schoene ML. Prolotherapy injections for chronic low-back pain. Cochrane Database of Systematic Reviews 2007, Issue 2. Art. No.: CD004059. DOI: 10.1002/14651858.CD004059.pub3

91   Ebadi S, Henschke N, Nakhostin Ansari N, Fallah E, van Tulder MW. Therapeutic ultrasound for chronic low-back pain. Cochrane Database of Systematic Reviews 2014, Issue 3. Art. No.: CD009169. DOI: 10.1002/14651858.CD009169.pub2

92   Sluka KA, Walsh D. Transcutaneous electrical nerve stimulation: basic science mechanisms and clinical effectiveness. J Pain. 2003;4(3):109–121.

93   Cheing GL, Hui-Chan CW. Transcutaneous electrical nerve stimulation: nonparallel antinociceptive effects on chronic clinical pain and acute experimental pain. Arch Phys Med Rehabil. 1999;80(3):305–312.

94   Deyo RA, Walsh NE, Martin DC, Schoenfeld LS,

Ramamurthy S. A controlled trial of transcutaneous electrical nerve stimulation (TENS) and exercise for chronic low back pain. N Engl J Med. 1990;322(23):1627–1634.

95   Jarzem PF, Harvey EJ, Arcaro N, Kaczorowski J. Transcutaneous electrical nerve stimulation (TENS) for chronic low back pain. J Musculoskelet Pain. 2005;13(2):3–9.

96   Topuz O, Özfidan E, Ozgen M, Ardic F. Efficacy of transcutaneous electrical nerve stimulation and percutaneous neuromodulation therapy in chronic low back pain. J Back Musculoskelet Rehabil. 2004;17(3–4):127–133.

97   Yousefi-Nooraie R, Schonstein E, Heidari K, et al. Low level laser therapy for nonspecific low-back pain. Cochrane Database of Systematic Reviews 2008, Issue 2. Art. No.: CD005107. DOI: 10.1002/14651858.CD005107.pub4

98   Furlan AD, Giraldo M, Baskwill A, Irvin E, Imamura M. Massage for low-back pain. Cochrane Database of Systematic Reviews 2015, Issue 9. Art. No.: CD001929. DOI:10.1002/14651858.CD001929.pub3

99   Cherkin DC, Sherman KJ, Kahn J, et al. A comparison of the effects of 2 types of massage and usual care on chronic low back pain: a randomized, controlled trial. Ann Intern Med. 2011 Jul;155(1):1–9.PubMed #21727288.
This study was analyzed by Paul Ingraham here: https://www.painscience.com/biblio/comparison-of-2-types-of-massage-for-chronic-low-back-pain.html

100   Furlan et al, op cit.

101   Steffens D, Maher CG, Pereira LS, et al. Prevention of Low Back Pain: A Systematic Review and Meta-analysis. JAMA Intern Med. 2016 Jan 11:1-10. doi: 10.1001/jamainternmed.2015.7431.

102   National Institute of Neurological Disorders and Stroke Low Back Pain Sheet: http://www.ninds.nih.gov/disorders/backpain/detail_backpain.htm

103   Lifting Safety: Tips to Help Prevent Back Injuries. http://familydoctor.org/familydoctor/en/prevention-wellness/staying-healthy/first-aid/lifting-safety-tips-to-help-prevent-back-injuries.html

104   Christensen ST1, Hartvigsen J. Spinal curves and health: a systematic critical review of the epidemiological literature dealing with associations between sagittal spinal curves and health. J

Manipulative Physiol Ther. 2008 Nov-Dec;31(9):690-714. doi: 10.1016/j.jmpt.2008.10.004.

105   Nourbakhsh MR1, Arab AM. Relationship between mechanical factors and incidence of low back pain. J Orthop Sports Phys Ther. 2002 Sep;32(9):447-60

106   Park S-D, Yu S-H. The effects of abdominal draw-in maneuver and core exercise on abdominal muscle thickness and Oswestry disability index in subjects with chronic low back pain. Journal of Exercise Rehabilitation. 2013;9(2):286-291. doi:10.12965/jer.130012.

107   Gokhale E. 8 Steps to a Pain-Free Back: Natural Posture Solutions for Pain in the Back, Neck, Shoulder, Hip, Knee, and Foot. Susan Adams: 9780979303609

108   http://www.webmd.com/sleep-disorders/excessive-sleepiness-10/pain-sleep

109   http://www.spine-health.com/wellness/sleep/chronic-pain-and-insomnia-breaking-cycle

110   Kovacs FM, Abraira V, Peña A, et al. Effect of firmness of mattress on chronic non-specific low-back pain: randomised, double-blind, controlled, multicentre trial. Lancet. 2003;362(9396):1599.

111   Derry S, Wiffen PJ, Moore RA, Quinlan J. Topical Lidocaine for Neuropathic Pain in Adults. In Cochrane Database of Systematic Reviews, edited by The Cochrane Collaboration. Chichester, UK: John Wiley & Sons, Ltd, 2014. http://doi.wiley.com/10.1002/14651858.CD010958.pub2.

112   Vad V. Back RX: A 15-Minute-a-Day Yoga- and Pilates-Based Program to End Low Back Pain: Hilary Hinzmann : 9781592400454:

113   Yip YB, Tse SHM. The effectiveness of relaxation acupoint stimulation and acupressure with aromatic lavender essential oil for non-specific low back pain in Hong Kong: a randomised controlled trial. Complementary Therapies in Medicine. 2004;12(1):28–37.

114   Sahar T, Cohen MJ, Ne'eman V, et al. Insoles for prevention and treatment of back pain. Cochrane Database of Systematic Reviews 2007, Issue 4. Art. No.: CD005275. DOI:10.1002/14651858.CD005275.pub2.

115   Steffens D, Maher CG, Pereira LS, et al. Prevention

of Low Back Pain: A Systematic Review and Meta-analysis. JAMA Intern Med. 2016 Jan 11:1-10. doi: 10.1001/jamainternmed.2015.7431.

116   Op cit, Sahar.

117   Elmasry S, Asfour S, de Rivero Vaccari JP, Travascio F. Effects of Tobacco Smoking on the Degeneration of the Intervertebral Disc: A Finite Element Study. PLoS ONE. 2015 10(8): e0136137. doi:10.1371/journal.pone.0136137 http://journals.plos.org/plosone/article?id=10.1371/journal.pone.0136137.

118   Goldberg MS1, Scott SC, Mayo NE. A review of the association between cigarette smoking and the development of nonspecific back pain and related outcomes. Spine (Phila Pa 1976). 2000 Apr 15;25(8):995-1014.

119   Holm S and Nachemson A. Nutrition of the intervertebral disc: acute effects of cigarette smoking—An experimental animal study. Upsala Journal of Medical Science. 1988 93: 91–99.

120   Uematsu Y, Matuzaki H, Iwahashi M. Effects of nicotine on the intervertebral disc: an experimental study in rabbits. Journal of Orthopaedic Science. 2001 6: 177–182. pmid:11484105 doi: 10.1007/s007760100067

121   Iwahashi M, Matsuzaki H, Tokuhashi Y, et al. Mechanism of intervertebral disc degeneration caused by nicotine in rabbits to explicate intervertebral disc disorders caused by smoking. Spine. 2002 27: 1396–1401. pmid:12131735 doi: 10.1097/00007632-200207010-00005

122   Oda H, Matsuzaki H, Tokuhashi Y, et al. Degeneration of intervertebral discs due to smoking: experimental assessment in a rat-smoking model. Journal of Orthopaedic Science. 2004 9: 135–141. pmid:15045541 doi: 10.1007/s00776-003-0759-y

123   Nemoto Y, Matsuzaki H, Tokuhasi Y, et al. Histological changes in intervertebral discs after smoking and cessation: experimental study using a rat passive smoking model. Journal of Orthopaedic Science. 2006 11: 191–197. pmid:16568393 doi: 10.1007/s00776-005-0987-4

124   Wang D, Nasto LA, Roughley P, Leme AS, et al. Spine degeneration in a murine model of chronic human tobacco smoker. Osteoarthritis and Cartilage. 2012 20: 896–905. doi: 10.1016/j.joca.2012.04.010. pmid:22531458

125   Garzillo MJ, Garzillo TA. Does obesity cause low back

pain? J Manipulative Physiol Ther. 1994 Nov-Dec;17(9):601-4.

126   Uribarri J, Woodruff S, Goodman S, et al. Advanced Glycation End Products in Foods and a Practical Guide to Their Reduction in the Diet. Journal of the American Dietetic Association, 110(6), 911–16.e12. http://doi.org/10.1016/j.jada.2010.03.018

127   Illien-Jünger S, Lu Y, Qureshi SA, et al. Chronic ingestion of advanced glycation end products induces degenerative spinal changes and hypertrophy in aging pre-diabetic mice. PLoS One. 2015 Feb 10;10(2):e0116625. doi: 10.1371/journal.pone.0116625. eCollection 2015.

128   Schwalfenberg, G. The Alkaline Diet: Is There Evidence That an Alkaline pH Diet Benefits Health? J Environ Public Health. 2012; 2012: 727630.
Published online 2011 Oct 12. doi: 10.1155/2012/727630
PMCID: PMC3195546

129   Sheetz DA. Caffeine and chronic back pain. Arch Phys Med Rehabil. 1997 Jul;78(7):786.

130   Barton J & Pretty J. What is the Best Dose of Nature and Green Exercise for Improving Mental Health? A Multi-Study Analysis. Environmental Science & Technology 2010 44 (10), 3947-3955
    DOI: 10.1021/es903183r

131   Park BJ, Tsunetsugu Y, Kasetani T, et al. The physiological effects of Shinrin-yoku (taking in the forest atmosphere or forest bathing): evidence from field experiments in 24 forests across Japan. Environ Health Prev Med. 2010 Jan;15(1):18-26. doi: 10.1007/s12199-009-0086-9.

132   Li Q, Morimoto K, Nakadai A, et al. Forest bathing enhances human natural killer activity and expression of anti-cancer proteins. Int J Immunopathol Pharmacol. 2007 Apr-Jun;20(2 Suppl 2):3-8.

133   Brown DK, Barton JL, Gladwell VF. Viewing Nature Scenes Positively Affects Recovery of Autonomic Function Following Acute-Mental Stress. Environmental Science & Technology. 2013;47(11):5562-5569. doi:10.1021/es305019p.

134   Gladwell VF, Brown DK, Wood C, et al. The great outdoors: how a green exercise environment can benefit all. Extreme Physiology & Medicine 2013;2:3

DOI: 10.1186/2046-7648-2-3

135   Lee I, Shiroma EJ, Lobelo F et al. Effect of physical inactivity on major non-communicable diseases worldwide: an analysis of burden of disease and life expectancy. The Lancet. 380(9838): 219-229

136   Claus A, Hides J, Moseley GL, Hodges P. Sitting versus standing: does the intradiscal pressure cause disc degeneration or low back pain? Journal of Electromyography and Kinesiology: Official Journal of the International Society of Electrophysiological Kinesiology. 2008 18(4), 550–558. http://doi.org/10.1016/j.jelekin.2006.10.011

137   Lally P, van Jaarsveld CHM, Potts HWW, Wardle J. How are habits formed: modelling habit formation in the real world. Euro J Soc Psychol. 2010;40:998–1009.

138   Boden SD1, Davis DO, Dina TS, et al. Abnormal magnetic-resonance scans of the lumbar spine in asymptomatic subjects. A prospective investigation. J Bone Joint Surg Am. 1990 Mar;72(3):403-8.

139   Olmarker K, Blomquist J, Strömberg J, et al. Inflammatogenic properties of nucleus pulposus. Spine. 1995 Mar 15; 20(6):665-9.

140   Goupille P, Jayson MI, Valat JP, Freemont AJ. Matrix metalloproteinases: the clue to intervertebral disc degeneration? Spine. 1998 Jul 15; 23(14):1612-26.

141   Atlas SJ, Keller RB, Chang Y, et al. Surgical and nonsurgical management of sciatica secondary to a lumbar disc herniation: five-year outcomes from the Maine Lumbar Spine Study. Spine (Phila Pa 1976). 2001 May 15; 26(10):1179-87.

142   Weber H. Lumbar disc herniation. A controlled, prospective study with ten years of observation. Spine. 1983 Mar; 8(2):131-40.

143   Roth, P. 2014. *The End of Back Pain: Access Your Hidden Core to Heal Your Body* (1 edition). New York: HarperOne, p. 175

144   https://www.flickr.com/photos/michael_teller/4420356767/in/photolist-7JBu4H

145   Johnsson KE, Rosén I, Udén A. The natural course of lumbar spinal stenosis. Clin Orthop Relat Res. 1992 Jun;(279):82-6.

146   Lee MJ, Dettori JR, Standaert CJ, et al. The natural history

of degeneration of the lumbar and cervical spines: a systematic review. Spine. 2012 Oct;37(22 Suppl):S18-30.

147   Xia XP, Chen HL, Cheng HB. Prevalence of adjacent segment degeneration after spine surgery: a systematic review and meta-analysis. Spine. 2013 Apr;38(7):597-608.

148   Martin BI, Mirza SK, Comstock BA et al. Reoperation rates following lumbar spine surgery and the influence of spinal fusion procedures. Spine. 2007 32(3), 382–387. http://doi.org/10.1097/01.brs.0000254104.55716.46

149   Donelson R1, McIntosh G, Hall H. Is it time to rethink the typical course of low back pain? PM R. 2012 Jun;4(6):394-401; quiz 400. doi: 10.1016/j.pmrj.2011.10.015. Epub 2012 Mar 3.

150   Deyo, Richard A., et al. "Overtreating chronic back pain: time to back off?." The Journal of the American Board of Family Medicine 22.1 (2009): 62-68.

57522013R00117

Made in the USA
Charleston, SC
15 June 2016